The Power of Clinical and Financial Metrics

Achieving Success
in Your Hospital

The Power of Clinical and Financial Metrics

*Achieving Success
in Your Hospital*

Steven Berger

ACHE Management Series
Health Administration Press

Chicago, Illinois

09   08   07   06   05   5   4   3   2   1

Library of Congress Cataloging-in-Publication Data

Berger, Steven H.
    The power of clinical and financial metrics : achieving success in your hospital
 / Steven Berger.
        p. ; cm.
      ISBN-13: 978-1-56793-239-3 (alk. paper)
      ISBN-10: 1-56793-239-8 (alk. paper)
        1. Hospital—Administration.   2. Hospital—Business management.
    3. Hospital—Personnel management.   4. Hospital—Quality control.
    I. Title: Achieving success in your hospital.   II. Title.
      [DNLM: 1. Hospital Administration—method.   2. Financial Management—
    method.   3. Patient Satisfaction.   4. Personnel Management—method.
    5. Quality Assurance, Health Care—standards. WX 150 B496p 2005]
    RA971.3.B466 2005
    362.1'068'8—dc22

                                                                    2004060906

The paper used in this publication meets the minimum requirements of American National Standard for Information Sciences—Permanence of Paper for Printed Library Materials, ANSI Z39.48-1984.⊗™

Acquisitions editor: Audrey Kaufman; Project manager: Jane C. Williams; Cover designer: Megan Avery

Health Administration Press
A division of the Foundation
    of the American College of
    Healthcare Executives
One North Franklin Street
Suite 1700
Chicago, IL 60606–4425
(312) 424–2800

Brief Contents

Detailed Contents

This book is dedicated to Barbara and the kids.
You make all things worthwhile.

Acknowledgments

WRITING A BOOK is hard. It takes a lot of time and effort to get it just right, not to mention time away from family, friends, business commitments, and hobbies. But it has its benefits too, like the opportunity to share information that can help others improve their ability to succeed.

My gratitude goes out to those who, over the years, have been good enough to stop what they were doing, if only for a moment, to give me advice and counsel. They have helped me improve my abilities. You are always in my thoughts, and I am fully aware of the positive impact you have had in my development as a businessman and a trainer.

I thank my business partners, Mary Grace Wilkus and Thomas Johnston, for helping to develop a business model for Healthcare Insights that has led (and will continue to lead) to the success of our enterprise. Our company supports the strategies put forth in this book, and the information and strategies here apply to management and leadership beyond the healthcare industry.

I thank my editors, Audrey Kaufman and Jane C. Williams, at Health Administration Press for their pursuit of the excellent outcome of this book. They diligently pored over the original manuscript and subsequent edited copies to ensure that the final product meets the highest standards of publishing. I am grateful for their dedication.

As always, I thank my family, who takes the brunt of my "away" time when I write. My wife Barbara and our children—Sam, Ben, Arlie, and Emmalee—have been very supportive of my writing efforts, although

I am aware that doing so is a struggle and that they would much rather spend time with me. I have great respect for their devotion to my writing pursuits, and I am extremely grateful to each of them.

Finally, acknowledging the readers of this book is important. The information and techniques offered here are only as good as the work that readers are willing to put in to achieve the successful outcomes possible with these concepts. Only the readers who engage in the practices presented here will make a difference. It is to you that I say, good luck and happy reading!

Introduction

MANAGING ANY COMPANY is hard. Managing the modern American hospital is really hard. Just think of dealing with a hospital's many stakeholders and their very different focus:

- Board of directors—governance and setting clinical and financial goals
- Senior administration—establishing and achieving clinical and financial targets
- Physicians and their leadership—providing care and monitoring clinical outcomes
- Middle managers—overseeing clinical and financial outcomes within their unit
- Frontline staff—doing whatever they are told to accomplish
- Patients—demanding great clinical care and results
- Bond holders—hoping to obtain financial returns
- Investment managers—making decisions to ensure financial stability
- Suppliers and trade vendors—negotiating for their own financial profit

Now think about the difficulty of achieving the goal of excellent care and a sustainable—no, a good—bottom line. In fact, it is important to define what "excellent care" and "good bottom line" are.

Defining the ideal clinical, quality, customer satisfaction, and financial results is not hard. Using the many metric indicators available in the healthcare industry is also not difficult. The challenging task is setting the goal and then implementing the actions to achieve that goal. This book highlights the issues related to establishing the proper goals and monitoring the outcomes in a way that is efficient, is effective, and adds value.

Today, many of the 5,800 or so hospitals in America are still managing by gut, not aware of the mass of information available to help them. Information is everywhere, and most of it is extremely useful. There is verified and validated information on outcomes from peer hospitals. There is information on quality, quantity, impact, and operation of the hospital from yesterday, today, and even tomorrow. There is information that shows hospitals how to develop their processes and procedures in a more practical, conclusive manner.

Hospitals have significant opportunities to improve. The indicators presented in this book are time tested and relate directly to the manner in which hospitals operate. If used properly, these indicators allow hospitals to show immediate and demonstrable improvements to their stakeholders.

Using metrics is not just another management fad. Indicators specifically measure the outcomes of the actions taken by administrators, directors, managers, and staff in their day-by-day work. Such results can then be compared to those achieved in other hospitals. The power and weight of indicators can best be seen through these comparisons, making such comments as "we are doing a good job" possible.

This book offers a number of strategies that can be immediately put to practical use by hospital management. At the end of every chapter, practical tips are given as well. The issues addressed here include the following:

- Why a hospital should become information driven
- How to present information so that it is effective and useful for better decision making
- What a best-practice hospital looks like, and what elements and indicators are needed to become one
- What elements and indicators are involved in a balanced scorecard, and how one is used to significantly improve outcomes

- How the Six Sigma methodology works, and what a hospital can do to adopt it
- What financial and clinical indicators a hospital can successfully use in its operations
- Why the adoption of an employee-based pay-for-performance model can help accelerate the development of an information-driven hospital

The techniques discussed in this book work, and they have worked for some of the most highly successful hospitals in America. Seven case studies on six concepts are presented, demonstrating why these hospitals chose to become more information driven and what steps they took to achieve this goal.

The techniques are not one-time fixes. If applied correctly, they become an integral part of the management practices employed at the hospital every day. They are not onerous, time consuming, or difficult, and they do change the way that the hospital will operate in the future. Rather than follow a process orientation, the information-driven hospital values results and establishes consequences, both positive and negative, that are dependent on the outcomes. This practice is very different from that employed by many hospitals today. An outcomes orientation will change the way hospital business is performed, and will do so for the better!

CHAPTER ONE

Basic Tenets of the Information-Driven Hospital

Pleasant Flats Medical Center is a 320-bed institution located in a growing community in the Southwest. It has a highly qualified board made up of prominent citizens who are pillars of the community. The hospital auxiliary is dedicated to its mission of supporting hospital operations while providing a number of fund-raising services throughout the year.

Although located in a delightful neighborhood, situated on a lovely campus, and surrounded on one side by a small lake and on the other by a grove of wildflowers, Pleasant Flats was not producing the kinds of financial results it was capable of generating. Additionally, its patient satisfaction and safety, clinical, quality, and financial outcomes were spotty. A particular problem for Pleasant Flats was that it was not reporting these key operation elements in a systematic, consistent, concise, and coordinated manner, which would have allowed the organization to determine if the outcomes were, in fact, acceptable to its board and senior administration.

Yet this lack of full reporting did not appear to be an issue at Pleasant Flats. Although they were receiving some information, members of the board were not asking the types of questions that would have pushed the administration to develop the types of reports needed to move the organization forward in a more effective and efficient way. The board just did not know what to ask, or why. Board members knew of the basic operations of the hospital, as described to them by the administrators, but many of them just did not have the time or experience to ask the particular questions that would have caused the administration to act differently.

Jon Taylor, Pleasant Flats's chief executive officer (CEO), is well respected and admired for his skills in keeping the board informed of the latest regulatory developments and fund-raising outcomes. However, a decline in the financial results in recent years had occurred, which Mr. Taylor characterized as a consequence of the 1997 Medicare Balanced Budget Act and poor stock-market performance in the early 2000s. Additionally, the board received some clinical and quality results on a regular basis, but those outcomes were not fully explained to them, thus limiting their ability to ask pertinent questions.

Here was a hospital with terrific staff, great location, and esteemed leadership, and yet it was not living up to, nor was even aware of, its potential. Pleasant Flats did not have the information that would help it determine how well (or badly) it was performing across a wide variety of indicators, including financial, clinical, patient satisfaction and safety, and quality. What little information it had was not being reported in a manner that would lead to improved decision making. It was not an information-driven hospital.

What is encouraging, however, for Pleasant Flats and other hospitals today is the fact that placing just a little emphasis on goal setting, monitoring, and reporting will turn a dream of being an information-driven hospital into a reality.

WHEN ADMINISTRATORS ADMINISTER and managers manage, what are they overseeing? When board members evaluate the success of the organization, what are they looking at? When patients determine how they were cared for, what are they assessing? When physicians examine, treat, and discharge their patients, how do they know if the clinical outcomes are acceptable?

Simple questions, hard answers. If the American hospital or health system is to achieve superior results, it needs to create a culture of accountability supported by a set of objectively determined goals, all of which are anchored by solidly established metrics. As presented throughout this book, dozens (in fact, hundreds) of acceptable and actionable metrics can be used at the organizational and departmental levels. Establishing and using these *objective metrics* will push the organization forward.

Over the broad expanse of the American hospital landscape, a pattern emerges—one of vast opportunities for unparalleled improvements. These opportunities encompass a wide range of activities that are common to the hospital environment but, in many organizations, have never been effectively measured, monitored, reviewed, or evaluated. Some hospitals and health systems have seen the light, seized the opportunities, and aggressively pursued the openings presented to them. These organizations have been at the forefront of a battle in the healthcare community to improve the clinical outcomes of their patients while maintaining bottom-line outcomes acceptable to the investment community, which has so much capital (i.e., bond debt) tied up in the industry.

The healthcare industry today is fighting hard to provide quality care, maintain its generally favorable customer perception, and deal with dramatically increased costs with less-than-acceptable revenue increases (in some cases, decreases). Cost increases come from the following factors:

- Staffing shortages, including among registered nurses, radiology technicians, respiratory therapists, and pharmacists, drive up salary costs by 5 to 8 percent per year.
- Staff benefits, including health insurance and pension, drive up benefit costs by 20 to 40 percent per year.
- Other insurances, including property, casualty, and professional liability (malpractice), drive up insurance costs by 20 to 150 percent per year.
- Supplies, including pharmaceuticals and patient-implantable devices (e.g., drug-eluting stents), drive up nonsalary costs by 12 to 40 percent per year.

Revenue increases have not kept pace with such significant growth in costs. The three major third-party payers—Medicare, Medicaid, and managed care—have pursued a path of minimal increases to their annual reimbursement rate. Each of these payers has its own challenges, and primary among these challenges is maintaining financial viability in the face of budgetary constraints. This is a difficult dilemma for these payers, considering that their beneficiaries are demanding better pharmaceutical benefits, access to a wider range of providers (i.e., hospitals, physicians, alternative medicine), and more freedom of choice without referrals. As a result, the payers' outlays to providers are minimized, which in turn leads to nominal increases in hospital revenue budgets. Coupled with these expense issues is the difficulty faced by hospital administrators in generating a meaningful financial return while maintaining superior patient satisfaction and clinical outcomes.

There are a large variety of ways in which boards and administrators along with their directors, managers, and staff can achieve superior results within the financial; clinical; quality; and patient, physician, and employee satisfaction areas. Many of these methods are not difficult to follow, primarily involving the utilization of techniques and, in some cases, tools that allow the organization to understand its outcomes objectively. To determine the areas to measure, the organization and its employees undergo a process, which begins with awareness and ends in significantly improved outcomes.

This chapter presents an overview of the information-driven hospital (IDH), introduces basic management techniques that can maximize the impact of the IDH, and offers 11 financial metrics and 1 financial operating metric designed to improve financial outcomes.

WHAT IS THE INFORMATION-DRIVEN HOSPITAL?

An information-driven hospital is an organization that uses a group of numbers (metric indicators), which represent key success factors, to set goals derived through benchmarks. The IDH monitors the outcomes of these goals and takes actions (consequences) based on the outcomes.

The development of appropriate goals allows the IDH to identify acceptable action plans for implementation. Then, the IDH is able to use techniques and tools to monitor the results and communicate them back to the managers and staff involved in the actions. Attention is paid to the details of the goals at hand rather than to the process used to generate the outcome.

Additionally, the IDH employs a "best practice" approach to setting goals, recognizing the work done and excellent outcomes achieved at peer facilities. Hospitals that adopt an information-driven orientation do the following:

- Employ benchmarking as a directional marker for goal setting.
- Develop accountability to ensure that the goals are met.
- Adopt consequences, both positive and negative, as an accountability response.
- Achieve outcomes far exceeding those reached by the average hospital.

BASIC MANAGEMENT PROCESS AND ITS APPLICATION

Hospitals have so much data. In most hospitals, a plethora of computer systems hold hundreds, even thousands, of data elements on financial and clinical matters. Thus, in any given year, data exist on tens (or hundreds) of thousands of patients across inpatient, outpatient, emergency, and ambulatory departments and on patients of physician practices.

This abundance of data is mind boggling, so much so that many hospitals have not been able to take the data and use them to make improvements to their processes and practices. Part of the problem is that the data can often be meaningless. *Random House Dictionary* (1993) defines *data* as "individual facts" and *information* as "knowledge communicated or received concerning a particular fact or circumstance, with this knowledge gained through study, communication, research, instruction." These definitions spell out to hospitals that they need to take their data and turn them into useful information, which in turn will help hospitals make rational and objective decisions that will have a better-than-average chance of being successful.

The best way to ensure the success of turning data into useful information is to employ the following five-step management process, which when followed accordingly will yield astonishing results:

1. Set appropriate goals.
2. Create action plans to achieve goals.
3. Implement action plans.
4. Monitor the results of the implementation.
5. Communicate the results to the affected parties (closing the feedback loop).

This process is so easy to list but apparently so hard to accomplish. Over the course of teaching hundreds of healthcare management courses (from 2000 through 2004), this author has polled class members regarding the results of this basic management process in their organizations. Findings from such unscientific polls are as follows.

Set Appropriate Goals

Take the example of a class of 100, consisting mostly of healthcare management personnel overseeing both financial and clinical areas. Starting with Step 1, the class is asked, "How many of you believe that your organization sets the right goals?" Generally, only 60 percent of hands go up for this question. This response immediately tells us that 40 percent of the managers and administrators in the class do not believe that their administration is appropriately setting goals for the organization. Even when the poll is repeated just moments after it is initially taken, for the sake of clarification, the same answer is given time and again. You may ask, "How can this be, especially when the same approximate answer is encountered in a class full of administrators?" We will come back to this question later.

Create Action Plans to Achieve Goals

Remember that 40 percent (or 40 people) of the class already believe that the first step in the management process has not been effectively achieved, leaving only 60 percent (or 60 people) of the original 100 class members to determine whether their organization can do Step 2—create action plans to achieve goals, which these 60 people believe have been appropriately set. Of the 60, generally 20 hands go down in response, leaving only 40 class members who believe that their organization not only sets appropriate goals but also creates action plans to achieve those goals. Within the first two steps of this basic five-step management process poll, we have already lost 60 percent of the group.

Implement Action Plans

When we pose the third question (regarding Step 3) to the remaining 40 class members—"How many of you believe that your organization implements the action plans that have been established?"—another 20 hands go down. This leaves just 20 percent of the original 100 who believe their organization has achieved success in the first three steps of the five-step process. Put another way, 80 percent of this class do not believe that these basic management techniques have been adopted by or achieved at their organization.

Monitor the Results of the Implementation

At this point, class members who believe that their organization effectively implements the action plans to achieve the appropriately set goals are near unanimous on agreeing that their organization continues to do an efficient job at Step 4—monitoring the results of the implementation. This response indicates that the reports being produced contain value-added information that allows the readers of these reports to make further decisions.

Communicate the Results to the Affected Parties

Finally, class members who believe that implementation results are being monitored in an appropriate manner also believe that these results are being effectively communicated back to the affected parties (Step 5). Again, only 20 percent of the original class members believe these five steps are being carried out.

These results, while unscientific, repeat themselves in poll after poll (see Figure 1.1). What can we say about these results? How can they be correct? Are they correct? If they are correct, what do they say about the hospital industry? These and other questions like them are the reason that this book has been written. These results are very representative of the state of the hospital industry today. The reality, according to many class members polled over the years, is that many hospitals *do not do the following:*

FIGURE 1.1 BASIC MANAGEMENT PROCESS POLL RESULTS

How many of you believe that your organization . . .

Sets appropriate goals	60%
And, creates action plans to achieve goals	40%
And, implements action plans	20%
And, monitors the results of the implementation	20%
And, communicates the results to the affected parties (closing the feedback loop)	20%

Note: The first question is asked of all class members. Subsequent questions are asked of those who answer affirmatively to the question before.
Source: Results based on unscientific classroom polls over a five-year period, from 2000 through 2004.

- Appropriately set objective goals in a systematic and serious manner.
- Regularly monitor these goals so that failure to meet the goals has significant negative consequences for the individual charged with responsibility for the goal.
- Consistently communicate the results of the actual outcomes back to the managers whose job it is to meet the goals.

IDHs operate differently from average hospitals. Through their utilization of metrics, based on time-tested indicators and peer-group numerical outcomes, IDHs are able to achieve results significantly better than institutions that do not.

THE IMPORTANCE OF METRICS

Hospitals have so many opportunities to improve their outcomes, and this effort *all starts with the numbers*—objectively developed metrics that are the backbone, the baseline, the heart of the matter. Metrics go by various names, many of them intuitive and others not. Figure 1.2 lists some of these alternative names.

The last term in Figure 1.2—truth—is perhaps the most evocative. Metrics is truth; metrics as truth! No more need for subjectivity, speculation, gut feeling, bias, prejudice, or partisanship. No more relying

FIGURE 1.2 ALTERNATIVE NAMES FOR METRICS

Analytics	Proof
Data	Reality
Details	Records
Essentials	Reporting
Evidence	Specifics
Facts	Statistics
Figures	Truth
Information	

on hearsay, gossip, or conjecture. Metrics allow the organization to operate on the truth (facts), with the truth (figures), and nothing but the truth (information). This is possible because the IDH has facts at hand—facts that were developed during the goal-setting process, honed throughout the action-plan creation, and adopted within the implementation phase. The IDH continuously updates its information with the knowledge gained in the measurement and monitoring stages, and this process periodically concludes during the feedback stage.

FINANCIAL METRICS: 11 KEY SUCCESS FACTORS

It is important to use metrics that have credibility within the healthcare industry, as these are metrics that have been accepted over time as having authority and influence. Eleven financial metrics have great significance to hospitals:

1. Operating margin
2. Excess margin
3. Debt service coverage
4. Current ratio
5. Cash on hand
6. Cushion ratio
7. Accounts receivable days
8. Average payment period
9. Average age of plant
10. Debt to capitalization
11. Capital expense

These metrics have been given weight within the industry by investors and their managers (generally, bond investors), bankers, academics, and government officials, and they are the first metrics reviewed by these stakeholders. Additionally, these metrics have been used and

Measure	S & P[1]	Fitch[2]	Solucient[3] (HBSI, HCIA)	Data Advantage Corp[4]	Ingenix[5]	Premier, Inc.[6]
Sample size (n)	577	215	779	4,424	1,753	380
Average length of stay (%)	4.6	4.7	4.73	4.8	5.01	4.68
Maintained bed occupancy (%)	64.3	N/A	67.33	63.07	51.1	67.3
Net patient revenue ($000)	200,846	289,791	164,956	95,072	47,007	47,365
Operating margin (%)	1.9	1.6	4.1	−0.58	0.69	2.54
Excess margin (%)	2.9	2.6	4.8	5.7	5.11	4.2
Debt service coverage (x)	2.9	2.8	4.51	N/A	2.94	N/A
Current ratio (x)	1.94	N/A	2.12	1.83	1.88	2.47
Cash on hand (days)	139.7	149.6	86.09	47.07*	64.1	N/A
Cushion ratio (%)	10.6	10.6	N/A	N/A	8.1	N/A
Accounts receivable (days)	54.5	54.2	53.43	58.81	59.3	54.81
Average payment period (days)	59.4	64.3	46.35	65.43*	48.1	N/A
Average age of plant (years)	9.5	9.5	N/A	8.78*	9.8	N/A
Debt to capitalization (%)	39.3	44.2	45.38	32.08	27.2	44
Capital expense (%)	7.4	N/A	6.69	6.64*	6.4	6.9

* Data for sample size of 699
1. Standard & Poor's Ratings Group, 2004 median healthcare ratios
2. FITCH, 2004 median ratios for nonprofit hospitals and health care systems
3. © 2004 Solucient, LLC ACTION O-I ™ Program (January–December 2003 median data)
4. Copyright 2004 by Data Advantage Corporation
5. © 2004 Ingenix, Inc., financial analysis and strategic operating indicators services and Medicare cost reports
6. Premier, Inc., operations outlook for the year ending June 30, 2004

Source: Healthcare Financial Management Association, Westchester, Illinois.

currently are being used every day by a number of hospitals to improve their financial outcomes. These metrics can and should be used to drive organizational goals.

Annually, the Healthcare Financial Management Association puts together a matrix that compares the performance on these 11 financial metrics among bond-rating agencies and major proprietary benchmarking systems (see Table 1.1).

These metrics are developed using an organization's balance sheet and statement of operations (income statement). To help readers gain an understanding of how metrics work, a balance sheet and an income statement have been created for this purpose (see Appendices 1.1 and 1.2). These two documents will be the basis for all of the organizational-level financial metrics that will be reviewed in this book.

Each of the metrics has its own unique features and applicability, providing the organization with information that can be reviewed and compared against budget, benchmark, stretch goal, and itself over time (trending).

A note of interest is in order here. Using all of these metrics means that the organization, generally for the first time, will be budgeting its balance sheet. Because many of these 11 metrics use balance-sheet numbers, setting goals around the metric means setting goals around the underlying line items. This is a very effective way to produce better balance-sheet results.

Table 1.2 defines and allows us to analyze Pleasant Flats's key financial metrics. Benchmark information on all of these metrics is readily available through bond-rating agencies and proprietary benchmarking services.

The Most Important Financial Operating Metric Today

The metrics defined in Table 1.2 are essential to understanding the financial health of hospitals. They allow readers of financial statements to determine how well the hospital is performing financially, and the metrics have been adopted by two bond-rating agencies—Standard & Poor's and Fitch. As such, they must all be used.

One metric available today will allow administrators to know instantly if they are operating efficiently, particularly in labor costs. This metric is generally known as *Salaries, Wages, Contract Labor, and Fringe Benefits as a Percentage of Total Revenues.*

TABLE 1.2 KEY FINANCIAL METRICS: DEFINITIONS AND EXAMPLES

Metric Name	Equation	What it Is	Importance of the Metric
Operating margin (Preferred direction of result: higher)	(Total operating revenues minus total operating expenses) divided by (total operating revenues)	This metric reflects the profit margin in relation to the *core operating revenues* of the organization. The goal should be to maximize the financial returns to the organization.	This is one of the most important financial metrics in this group, according to the bond-rating agencies. It allows the evaluator to determine, by percentage, how effectively the healthcare organization is able to operate financially for the time period in question. This operating "bottom line" is often the only number many readers get to see.

Operating margin

$$\frac{\$ -1{,}200 \text{ Operating margin}}{\$ 96{,}700 \text{ Total operating revenues}}$$

Actual	Budget	Benchmark
−1.2%	4.0%	1.5%

Metric Name	Equation	What it Is	Importance of the Metric
Excess margin (Preferred direction of result: higher)	(Total operating revenues minus total operating expenses plus nonoperating revenues) divided by (total operating revenues)	This metric reflects the profit margin in relation to the *total overall revenues* of the organization. The goal should be to maximize the financial returns to the organization.	The excess margin reflects the total "bottom line" of the organization—operating margin plus nonoperating revenues. Nonoperating revenues include investment income (or losses) on excess cash and marketable securities. This allows the reader to determine the overall profitability of the organization.

Excess margin

$$\frac{\$ 6{,}400 \text{ Net margin}}{\$ 96{,}700 \text{ Total operating revenues}}$$

Actual	Budget	Benchmark
6.6%	6.0%	2.0%

Debt service coverage (Preferred direction of result: higher)	(Excess of revenues over expenses plus depreciation plus interest expense) divided by (principal plus interest payments)	This is one of the three debt ratios. It is often used by rating agencies and others to determine the hospital's ability to meet its long-term principal and interest obligations on a year-by-year basis. Current bond ratings are determined by the quality of this metric.

Debt service margin

$$\frac{\$24{,}800 \text{ Operating margin} + \text{depreciation} + \text{interest}}{\$10{,}900 \text{ Principal} + \text{interest expense}}$$

Actual	Budget	Benchmark
2.28	3.2	3.2

Current ratio (Preferred direction of result: higher)	Current assets divided by current liabilities	This metric measures the organization's ability to pay off (meet) its current financial responsibilities with its current assets. The goal should be to have at least twice the current assets as current liabilities. This is typically achieved through bottom-line maximization.	Every organization wants to ensure that it has enough liquid assets to pay off its current liabilities, which include payroll and trade vendor expenses as well as capital expenditures. The current ratio gives the reader a good sense of the organization's capabilities in meeting its current obligations.

Current ratio

$$\frac{\$24{,}800 \text{ Current assets}}{\$19{,}500 \text{ Current liabilities}}$$

Actual	Budget	Benchmark
1.27	1.50	2.00

(continued on following page)

TABLE 1.2 (continued)

| Days cash on hand —all sources (Preferred direction of result: higher) | (Unrestricted cash and investments) divided by [(average daily cash-operating requirements) defined as (total expenses) minus (depreciation and amortization expense) divided by (365)] | This metric represents the organization's ability to meet its short-term obligations and long-term capital-replacement needs. The goal should be to maximize the cash balances. This is typically achieved through bottom-line maximization and accounts-receivable minimization. | According to the bond-rating agencies, this is the *most important* financial metric because it measures how much cash the organization has to pay off both its current and long-term obligations, particularly any bond debt out-standing. The greater the cash balances, the greater the flexibility an organization has in making hard decisions about its future. Lower cash balances indicate less flexibility and less ability to meet its financial obligations. |

Days cash on hand

$ 103,200 Unrestricted cash and investments

$ 238.1 Average daily cash operating requirements ((97,900–11,000) / 365)

Actual	Budget	Benchmark
433.5	440.0	160.0

| Cushion ratio (Preferred direction of result: higher) | (Unrestricted cash and investments) divided by maximum annual debt service (MADS) [defined as annual depreciation and interest expense] | This metric represents the relationship between available cash and total debt service and is one of the three debt ratios. The goal should be to maximize the organization's cash balances so that they can offset any annual debt service obligations. | This is one of three important debt ratios. It allows us to determine if cash levels are high enough to meet debt obligations. For example, a value of 9 suggests that the organization has cash reserves 9 times its annual debt obligation. This is typically achieved through higher margins and cash management. |

Cushion ratio

$ 103,200 Unrestricted cash and investments

$ 10,900 Principal and interest expense

Actual	Budget	Benchmark
9.5	9.7	9.8

| Days in accounts receivable (Preferred direction of result: lower) | Net receivable divided by (average net daily revenue) [based on 90-day rolling average or annual financial statement information] | This metric represents the amount of net revenue dollars tied up in the hospital's accounts receivable. It is a proxy for the efficiency of the revenue cycle management. The goal should be to minimize the total receivables through exceptional revenue cycle management. This is typically achieved through the use of specific revenue cycle metrics (discussed in later chapters). | Most hospital analysts list this metric as critical to proper financial management functioning. It is usually reported as the one metric to describe the results of the revenue cycle. Benchmark information is readily available but should be viewed as a direction, rather than an absolute goal, because of the various assumptions within the metric—particularly payer mix—built into the ratio. | Actual 63.3 | Budget 60.0 | Benchmark 57.6 |

Days in accounts receivable

$$\frac{\$16,200,000 \text{ Net receivable}}{\$255,890 \text{ Average daily net receivable}} \quad (93,400,000/365 \text{ days})$$

(continued on following page)

TABLE 1.2 (continued)

Metric	Formula	Description	Additional Notes
Average payment period in days (Preferred direction of result: lower)	Current liabilities divided by average daily cash operating expenses	This metric measures the length of time the organization takes to pay its current bills. The goal should be to pay all current liabilities within the terms of the contract. This is typically achieved through bottom-line maximization and payment policies that stress paying obligations on time.	Credit-rating agencies are very concerned with the quality of the organization's result of this metric. Longer-than-average payment periods can negatively affect bond ratings and trade vendor credit terms.

Average payment period (days)

$$\frac{\$\,19,500,000 \text{ Current liabilities}}{\$\,238,082 \text{ (Total expenses--depreciation)}/365}$$

Actual	Budget	Benchmark
81.9	65.0	65.0

Metric	Formula	Description	Additional Notes
Average age of plant (Preferred direction of result: lower)	Accumulated depreciation divided by annual depreciation expense	This metric measures the equivalent age of the organization's fixed assets. It relates the accumulated depreciation of all the fixed assets currently on the plant ledger to the level of total current depreciation expense. The goal should be to achieve the lowest result, which represents a younger and thus more competitive plant. This is achieved through higher capital spending.	This is quite possibly the most underrated financial metric. It is very easy to compute and, when compared to the benchmark, allows the organization to measure the relative age of its facilities and equipment. This metric can be used as a major factor in determining the amount of the organization's current-year capital budget.

Average age of plant

$$\frac{\$\,72,000,000 \text{ Accumulated depreciation}}{\$\,11,000,000 \text{ Depreciation expense}}$$

Actual	Budget	Benchmark
6.55	7.00	9.50

| Debt-to-capitalization percentage (Preferred direction of result: lower) | (Long-term debt plus capital leases minus current maturities) divided by (long-term debt plus capital leases minus current maturities plus unrestricted net assets) | This metric measures the level of debt that the organization is carrying compared to its unrestricted net assets. Higher values indicate a higher level of debt financing and possibly a decreased ability to carry additional debt. This may be justifiable depending on the use of the debt. | This is one of the three debt ratios. This is one debt ratio most often used by bond investors and rating agencies to determine the organization's ability to repay its long-term obligations. It is proxy for determining how much the organization has leveraged its balance sheet for the level of its debt. |

Debt-to-capitalization percentage

$\dfrac{\$ 116{,}500{,}000 \text{ Long term debt–current maturities}}{\$ 186{,}400{,}000 \text{ Long term debt–current maturities + unrestricted net assets}}$

Actual	*Budget*	*Benchmark*
62.5%	60.0%	41.9%

| Capital expenses percentage (Preferred direction of result: trend is more important than direction) | Interest expenses plus depreciation expenses divided by total expenses times 100 | This metric measures the annual expenses related to the acquisition of fixed assets as a percentage of total expenses. Assuming the organization wants to minimize its average age-of-plant ratio, the goal should be to maximize its annual capital purchases, thus increasing its depreciation expense. | Recognizing that this ratio can be affected by many variables, it is important for the organization to review the numerator and denominator to maximize the outcomes. |

Capital expenses percentage

$\dfrac{\$ 18{,}700 \text{ Interest + depreciation}}{\$ 96{,}700 \text{ Total expenses}}$

Actual	*Budget*	*Benchmark*
19.34	19.00	6.80

Review the statement of operations in Appendix 1.2 (page 22). Take the already combined items of $50 million in Salary and Benefit Expenses and divide that amount by the $96.7 million of Total Revenues. The result is 51.7 percent. By itself, this percentage has no meaning, but when compared with peer information, 51.7 percent takes on significant meaning. For example, over the past several years, Fitch— one of the three well-known bond-rating agencies—has presented this metric in its annual review of the hospital industry. The median percentages of all of Fitch's rated hospitals (in reports published in 2002, 2003, and 2004) were 51.2 percent, 52.0 percent, and 52.2 percent. With this information, it becomes easy to see that Pleasant Flats, at 51.7 percent, is performing better than the overall median. That is good news for the organization.

Consider this, however. Over the past several decades, the largest for-profit hospital provider, HCA, which currently owns approximately 200 hospitals, has consistently reported its personnel costs at 40 percent of total revenues, a difference of more than 12 percentage points in 2004 and a consistent difference at that. How is it that HCA is able to use only 40 percent of its revenues for staffing expenses, while the Fitch median hospitals are at 52.2 percent? A number of reasons explain this difference, but essentially it comes down to this: HCA understands the importance of this metric, sets goals around it, and expects its managers to meet those goals. Many not-for-profit hospitals are not aware of the metric and therefore cannot set the appropriate goals, which would be lower than the median.

This is the most important financial operating metric in hospitals today because it has such a dramatic impact on the bottom lines of organizations. Just setting a goal around this one metric will change the way a hospital operates, forcing it to make staffing decisions that directly affect operations. Knowing that a peer hospital system is able to achieve financial outcomes far exceeding its own can help an organization to ask the right questions about its own operations.

The 11 financial metrics along with the 1 financial operating metric described in this chapter give administrators an objective picture of their financial health compared to that of their peers. This understanding is considerably important in setting financial goals and establishing plans of action to achieve superior results. These metrics are the backbone of the IDH.

Jon Taylor had not yet heard about these 11 financial metrics, having been more focused on the patient satisfaction area that the Joint Commission on Accreditation of Healthcare Organizations had mandated to be reported on a periodic basis. Although he found it somewhat onerous to have to report on the numbers each month, he had not yet recognized that the 52nd percentile that Pleasant Flats was running in the total satisfaction category gave the organization an opportunity to differentiate itself from the other hospital in town. He had not yet determined that setting the goal at the 90th, 95th, or 99th percentile was the first step in a process of dramatic improvement, able to be accomplished in a short period of time (that is, under a year).

His old notions were about to change.

REFERENCE

Random House Dictionary. 1993. New York: Random House Reference.

PRACTICAL TIPS

☞ Develop a presentable and reproducible report with the 11 financial metrics. Set up the report to include *month* and *year to date* for the following:
  1. Prior-year actual
  2. Current actual
  3. Current budget
  4. Variances
☞ Also consider adding a stretch-goal column, giving leadership and management additional goals to achieve.
☞ Pick one or two of the 11 metrics that the organization believes need to be improved, and develop specific plans for improvement. Set time limits, and identify the individuals who will be responsible for achieving the goals. After initial achievement, adopt goals for all other financial metrics.

ASSETS:

Current assets

	December	
	2004	2003
Cash	$1,200	$2,000
Investments—short term	6,500	5,400
Total cash and cash equivalents	7,700	7,400
Accounts receivable	27,000	27,800
Less: Allowance for contractual adjustments	(5,000)	(5,000)
Less: Allowance for doubtful accounts	(5,800)	(5,600)
Net patient receivables	16,200	17,200
Inventory	500	400
Prepaid expenses	400	300
Other current assets:	900	700
Total current assets	24,800	25,300

LIABILITIES:

Current liabilities

	December	
	2004	2003
Accounts payable and accrued liabilities	$12,000	$10,000
Third-party liabilities	4,000	4,500
Current retirement on long-term debt	3,500	3,400
Total current liabilities	19,500	17,900
Long-term debt	120,000	123,400
Other long-term liabilities	4,000	4,100
Total long-term liabilities	124,000	127,500
Total Liabilities	$143,500	$145,400

Long-term investments—unrestricted	$ 95,500	$ 87,000
Trusteed investments	22,000	30,000
Endowment fund investments	300	300
Deferred financing costs	3,300	3,400
Other noncurrent assets	121,100	120,700
Property, plant, and equipment (PP&E)		
Land and land improvements	8,000	7,000
Buildings	70,000	60,000
Leasehold improvements	3,000	2,800
Equipment and fixtures	56,000	51,600
Construction in progress	3,000	4,000
Total PP&E	140,000	125,400
Less: Accumulated depreciation	(72,000)	(61,000)
Net PP&E	68,000	64,400
Total assets	213,900	210,400
NET ASSETS:		
Unrealized gain/(loss) on investments	$ 2,000	$ 3,000
Unrestricted	67,900	61,500
Temporarily restricted	200	200
Permanently restricted	300	300
Total Net Assets	70,400	65,000
Total Liabilities and Net Assets	213,900	210,400

	2004	2003	Percentage Change
REVENUES:			
Inpatient revenue	$73,000	$74,000	−1.35
Outpatient revenue	72,000	69,000	4.35
Total patient revenue	145,000	143,000	1.40
Less:			
Contractual and other adjustments	(49,000)	(48,000)	2.08
Charity care	(2,600)	(2,200)	18.18
Net patient service revenue	93,400	92,800	0.65
Add:			
Other operating income	3,300	2,500	32.00
Total revenue	96,700	95,300	1.47
EXPENSES:			
Salaries	42,000	40,000	5.00
Contract labor	1,000	1,500	−33.33
Fringe benefits	7,000	6,800	2.94
Total salaries and benefits	50,000	48,300	3.52
Patient care supplies	11,500	11,000	4.54
Professional and management fees	3,600	3,600	0.00
Purchased services	7,200	8,800	−18.18
Operation of plant (including utilities)	2,600	2,500	4.00
Depreciation	11,000	10,500	4.76
Interest and financing expenses	7,400	7,600	−2.63
Bad debts	4,600	4,400	4.55
Total expenses	97,900	96,700	1.24
Operating margin	(1,200)	(1,400)	−14.29
NONOPERATING INCOME:			
Gain/(loss) on investments	1,200	600	100.00
Investment income	6,400	5,500	16.36
Total nonoperating income	7,600	6,100	24.59
Net income	6,400	4,700	36.17

CHAPTER TWO

Presenting Metrics to Produce the Greatest Operational Impact

Like many hospitals throughout the United States, Pleasant Flats oper-ated by gut feel—a seat-of-the-pants type of management that permits a substantially wide variety of outcomes, both financial and clinical. Although these hospitals purportedly have to meet or exceed goals that have been established by the board of directors, they face two realities: (1) generally the goals are not set with any objective factors in mind and (2) after the goals are set, they are not always monitored well or followed through by the board.

Having attended a seminar on better reporting techniques, Pleasant Flats's board chair, Zeke Brown, asked the CEO, Jon Taylor, to reevaluate the board reporting and monitoring systems currently in place and to suggest improvements to the process. Jon was somewhat baffled by the request, given that he had been reporting information to the board for 22 years and was very comfortable with the process. Still, he turned to his CFO, Jane Zabrowsky, to identify the "problem" and to report back to him with potential solutions.

Jane has been the CFO at Pleasant Flats for the past three years. Prior to her current role, she was assistant CFO at a slightly smaller hospital on the other side of town. She was intrigued by the board chair's request, as she also had been thinking of revamping the current reporting methods. Over the past six months or so, Jane had been thinking that the organization could be doing better, but part of the problem appeared to be the reporting structure, which was shielding many of the poor performers from detection.

At the present time, the board (and administration) was receiving a 30-page monthly report, the format of which was developed before Jane's tenure. A lot of information was reported for no apparent reason. At the monthly meeting of the board's finance committee, only five pages of the entire report were actually reviewed; the rest were deemed to be "for information only," except that there were so many for-information-only pages that Jane believed they could not be accessible to the board members.

Also, often, no conclusion or narrative was given to the information reported. Jane was disturbed that conclusions, such as action plans for improvements, were not part of the reports. She had prepared different reports at her previous hospital that included actionable elements. In the past, when she discussed with Jon the tweaking of the current reporting system, he said, "Listen, this is how we have been doing this for a long time, and successfully I might add. I am not looking to make any changes at this time. The board is happy. I am happy. Leave it alone."

In complying with the board chair's request, Jane wanted to be sure that she accomplished a number of goals, including the following:

a. Decide whether the current 30-page report was meeting the needs of the board and administration.
b. Determine the types of reporting methods available to Pleasant Flats.
c. Establish an outcomes-based action plan to ensure improvements in reporting and monitoring.

Little did Jane know that she was taking on a project that would not only reshape the look of the reports but also would have extremely positive effects on the future outcomes of Pleasant Flats.

THE REPORTS GENERATED by financial, information technology, and clinical analysts within a hospital or healthcare system do not provide the information necessary for general management and leadership functions to be carried out. This finding is based on responses to the question, "While working in a hospital, have you *ever* produced a requested report that you knew, even as you were creating it, would be useless?" This question is put forth in every class by this author, and more than 90 percent of the class raise their hand to acknowledge they have done so (the rest seem to be in denial).

Why do managers create a report that they know will not be useful? The obvious answer is that they were asked to do so by their bosses. That answer, however, simply advances the problems inherent with the hospital reporting process. Why would anyone ask for reports that they will find useless and not use? How did we get to this stage? More importantly, how can we correct this?

Specific actions can be taken by any hospital to immediately improve its report creation and generation practices. The first step is to recognize that information can be used within all segments of a hospital's operation to enhance revenue, reduce expenses, improve customer service, strengthen clinical outcomes, and increase quality indicators. Other benefits include the following:

- Improved communication inside and outside the organization
- Enhanced ability to produce more reasonable planning and forecasting
- Increased productivity
- Greater efficiency in all aspects of the operation

THE TEN ELEMENTS OF GOOD REPORTING

Hospitals have an opportunity to substantially enhance the effectiveness of their reporting to access all of these improvements. They need only to apply the ten elements of good reporting every time. The ten elements are listed in Figure 2.1. They represent an absolute test for determining whether a report will be effective to the recipient or decision maker.

The elements in Figure 2.1 appear innocuous, basic, and easy to apply. However, across time, across hospitals, and across practice, most reports in fact do not meet all ten elements. If the report designer applies these elements, the report reader will certainly be able to *render a decision* based on the content of the report. It is a truism that the only reason to generate/create/produce a report is so that an action may be taken based on the information. Put another way, taking the time to produce a report is senseless unless *the report leads to an action plan*. If you are a decision maker, do not ask for a report you do not plan to use, as the report designer's time can be used better in creating other actionable reports. If you are a report designer, first ascertain

FIGURE 2.1 TEN ELEMENTS OF GOOD REPORTING

In all events, reports should be

1. Useful, as determined by the user
2. Relevant, as determined by the user
3. Understandable, or clear
4. Straightforward, not overly complicated
5. Inclusive, including comparative information
6. Attractive, or easy on the eye
7. Accurate, with sources that are verifiable
8. Timely, keeping in mind that one day after deadline is too late
9. Cost effective, with report benefits exceeding the cost
10. Filled with narrative, including a short blurb from the analyst

how the report is going to be used, again as your time should not be wasted. If both parties adhere to this rule, the organization can see the following differences:

- More effective reports that lead to better decisions
- Better decisions that lead to improved outcomes (e.g., financial, clinical, customer satisfaction)
- Improved outcomes that lead to higher compensation for all
- Higher compensation that leads to greater satisfaction with reporting
- Greater reporting satisfaction that leads to even more effective reporting

Later in the chapter a number of sample reports will be reviewed to determine if each meets the ten elements. Then, each report will be classified as good, bad, or ugly—terms that will be defined later.

The Design of a Useful Report

The first two prime elements of good reporting are *useful* and *relevant*. Usefulness and relevance must be determined by the report reader—the decision maker—not by the report designer. The report designer's first,

FIGURE 2.2 QUESTIONS TO ENSURE USEFULNESS OF REPORTS

- Who is the recipient of the report?
- With whom does the reader plan to share the report?
- What is the purpose or objective of the report?
- What kinds of information should be included to satisfy this purpose or objective?
- What time periods should the report cover?
- How often should the report be generated?
- What is the reporting medium—paper, electronic? What should the report include—illustration, words?
- What decisions are we expecting to make with the reporting outcomes (benefits)?

second, and third thoughts always need to be focused on generating a report that is actionable to the reader, not convenient to the designer.

Figure 2.2 lists several questions that the designer must ask the reader so that a report is created appropriately and not wasted. Using this questionnaire can be designed to ensure that the report includes necessary information as requested by the reader.

Figure 2.3 is an example of such a questionnaire that can and should be used by designers when a new report is requested. The questionnaire will help the designer achieve reporting success every time. The answers to the questions will allow the designer to gain a complete understanding of the report users' needs. Thus, the designer can incorporate into the requested report the information deemed useful and relevant by the reader.

Figure 2.4 is an example of a completed questionnaire, which gives us a look at how the questionnaire works. In this particular example, the primary requestor and recipients of the report are identified (see responses 2 and 3). Response 4 sets the purpose for the new report: the director is interested in learning the amount of actual capacity available in the department to determine whether or not capital dollars are needed to expand the department, given the current waiting list for its services. The director plans to share the results with her boss and the affected clinicians.

Having established the purpose, the designer, along with the recipient, can now determine the types of elements needed to complete the

FIGURE 2.3 EXAMPLE QUESTIONNAIRE FOR NEW REPORT
DEVELOPMENT

1. Report name   _____

2. Primary recipient(s)   _____

3. Secondary recipient(s) _____

4. Report purpose   _____

    _____

5. Financial/nonfinancial elements that will satisfy the purpose

    _____

    _____

6. Source of the elements (Which computer system? Which fields?)

    _____

    _____

7. Frequency of reporting

    _____

8. Time period the report needs to cover_____

9. Expected decisions to be made from the report outcomes (benefits)

    _____

    _____

    _____

report and where these elements will come from (responses 5 and 6). In this case, as is often true in other cases, the source of the data, which will be turned into information, is partly manual. This concept needs to be emphasized: the data needed to develop a value-added report do not always come from an automated source. Data that will give the reader the information to achieve his or her purpose must be captured, regardless of the source.

Response 7 reflects the requestor's desire regarding the frequency with which the report is generated. Answers to question 7 will be different for each requested report, depending on the purpose. In this

FIGURE 2.4 EXAMPLE OF A COMPLETED QUESTIONNAIRE

1. Report name: <u>Capacity status of rehabilitation services</u>
2. Primary recipient(s): <u>Department director</u>
3. Secondary recipient(s): <u>Rehabilitation clinicians, vice president of professional services</u>
4. Report purpose: <u>To determine the actual available capacity in the department compared to the actual patients seen in the department to identify any unused capacity</u>
5. Financial/nonfinancial elements that will satisfy the purpose:
   a. <u>Available capacity by location</u>
   b. <u>Actual usage (billable units) by location</u>
   c. <u>Clinician productivity</u>
6. Source of the elements (Which computer system? Which fields?)
   a. <u>Manual</u>
   b. <u>Legacy HIS system</u>
   c. <u>Manual</u>
7. Frequency of reporting? <u>Weekly</u>
8. Time period the report needs to cover: <u>Previous three months, then ongoing</u>
9. Expected decisions to be made from the report outcomes (benefits):
   a. <u>Use the information to determine</u>
      i. <u>Whether there is a capacity problem</u>
      ii. <u>Why there is a waiting list</u>
      iii. <u>How to minimize/eliminate the waiting list (without capital expenditures)</u>

case, the director wishes to have a reviewable report on a weekly basis to determine the capacity issue. Other directors, on the other hand, may want to see this report daily, biweekly, monthly, or even quarterly. However, this frequency decision is up to the recipient. Response 8 states the recipient's preference regarding the time period the report will cover. In our example, the director would like to see information in weekly increments and covering the past three months and ongoing.

Finally, question 9 is essential, needing to be answered appropriately if the report is to have any meaning and usefulness. The response to this question allows the recipient to determine the appropriate decisions that need to be made.

Capacity Status for the Week Ending March 13, 2005

| | Actual | | Variances | | |
	Capacity*	Units Billed	Number	Percentage	Clinician Productivity
Date					
3/7/05	86	90	4	4.7	101%
3/8/05	92	80	−12	−13.0	93%
3/9/05	110	100	−10	−9.1	92%
3/10/05	87	86	−1	−1.1	94%
3/11/05	90	92	−2	−2.2	93%
3/12/05	40	32	−8	−20.0	84%
3/13/05	40	28	−12	−30.0	79%
Total	545	508	−37	−6.8	90%

* Number of clinical staff working this week multiplied by number of hours the location is open to service patients

The Result

With the information shown in Figure 2.4, the designer can now create a new, useful report. Table 2.1 illustrates such a report. In our example, the report is developed for the director of rehabilitation services to compare the actual available capacity against the actual patients seen to determine whether there is any unused capacity in the department. The director feels that the current waiting list is about to undermine the department's productivity, and she needed information for decision making.

The designer worked with the director to create the report, which is reflected in Figure 2.4 (the input). Table 2.1 (the output) is the result of this collaboration, arrayed in a format that meets the director's needs. With the designer asking the director the nine questions in Figure 2.3, the report's format took shape in *eight minutes*, allowing the director to approve (or modify, if appropriate) it on the spot. Afterward, the designer can take the approved design back to his or her office to build the actual report that will be reproduced in an ongoing manner on a weekly basis.

The design methodology using the nine questions is effective, and it allows the requested report to be useful and relevant to the reader or recipient every time.

REPORTS: THE GOOD, THE BAD, THE UGLY

To illustrate the other eight elements of good reporting (and revisit the first two described above), we will analyze sample reports and assess whether they have met the ten criteria. If not, we will classify them as ugly or bad. Examples of good reports will also be given later in the chapter.

The Ugly and The Bad: Sample Report 1

Take a look at Table 2.2 for example. So many things are wrong with this report (which we will refer to as Report 1) that it is not only ugly, it is also bad.

An ugly report is one that does not draw the eyes of the reader to the information or data. Such a report always includes too much data on the page, leaving the reader slogging his or her way through the morass. The designer of such a report is so concerned about including so much information that he or she failed to consider the readability or usability of the data presented. Many report designers subscribe to the unfortunate practice of "when in doubt, more is better." However, in almost all cases, the principle should be "when in doubt, less is better."

This report also displays a lot of bad elements (the opposite of the good elements), including the following:

- Not useful
- Not relevant
- Not understandable
- Not straightforward
- Not inclusive
- Not timely
- Not cost effective
- Not filled with narrative

Report 1 is bad on all accounts, except accuracy. Starting with usefulness and relevance, again, the nine questions have to be answered so that an understanding is gained of why the report has to be generated

COST CENTER	PP 24 OT HOURS WORKED	YTD OT HOURS WORKED	PP24 TOTAL HOURS WORKED	YTD TOTAL HOURS WORKED	PP24 % OF OVERTIME	YTD % OF OVERTIME
Patient Care Services – 1000	2.00	25.00	679.00	17697.00	0.29%	0.14%
Nursing Education – 101	5.00	75.00	199.00	4003.00	2.51%	1.87%
Nursing Float – 102	0.00	10.00	107.00	2590.00	0.00%	0.39%
Case Management – 103	17.00	46.00	98.00	2720.00	17.35%	1.69%
3 East – 1111	12.00	1258.00	1847.00	40066.00	0.65%	3.14%
3 Southwest – 1112	35.00	1544.00	1721.00	31074.00	2.03%	4.97%
3 Northeast – 1113	21.00	1754.00	1597.00	34987.00	1.31%	5.01%
Labor and Delivery – 1200	117.00	4247.00	3109.00	69993.00	3.76%	6.07%
Skilled Nursing Facility – 1300	68.00	3980.00	2520.00	58124.00	2.70%	6.85%
Inpatient Psychiatric – 1400	84.00	1092.00	2058.00	46474.00	4.08%	2.35%
Eating Disorder – 1401	4.00	15.00	287.00	7034.00	1.39%	0.21%
Day Treatment – 1402	0.00	7.00	417.00	7700.00	0.00%	0.09%
Surgery – 1500	32.00	634.00	2197.00	51375.00	1.46%	1.23%
Post Acute Care Unit – 1501	16.00	488.00	509.00	10984.00	3.14%	4.44%
Same Day Surgery – 1502	55.00	1039.00	735.00	16587.00	7.48%	6.26%
Outpatient Treatment Center – 1503	40.00	882.00	1358.00	29761.00	2.95%	2.96%
Emergency Department – 1600	168.00	4631.00	1915.00	43367.00	8.77%	10.68%
Emergency Medical Services – 1601	13.00	27.00	341.00	5502.00	3.81%	0.49%
Renal Dialysis – 1700	35.00	1046.00	1323.00	29403.00	2.65%	3.56%
Home Health Services – 1800	12.00	576.00	2924.00	62642.00	0.41%	0.92%
Hospice – 1801	8.00	103.00	241.00	7590.00	3.32%	1.36%

Department						
Adult Day – 1802	0.00	1.00	284.00	6895.00	0.00%	0.01%
Eye Center – 1803	1.00	87.00	81.00	2807.00	1.23%	3.10%
Home Health Services Administration – 1804	12.00	100.00	282.00	5635.00	4.26%	1.77%
Clinical Services Administration – 2000	0.00	5.00	80.00	2478.00	0.00%	0.20%
Women's Health Services – 2100	1.00	22.00	80.00	735.00	1.25%	2.99%
Lactation – 2101	8.00	91.00	111.00	2755.00	7.21%	3.30%
Physical Medicine and Rehabilitation – 2200	37.00	818.00	1921.00	46265.00	1.93%	1.77%
Speech Therapy – 2201	0.00	38.00	98.00	2288.00	0.00%	1.66%
Occupational Therapy – 2202	1.00	165.00	412.00	11530.00	0.24%	1.43%
EMG – 2300	3.00	17.00	102.00	1883.00	2.94%	0.90%
EEG – 2301	0.00	1.00	20.00	460.00	0.00%	0.22%
Cardiology – 2400	32.00	777.00	385.00	8351.00	8.31%	9.30%
Cardiac Rehabilitation – 2401	0.00	30.00	402.00	8922.00	0.00%	0.34%
Cardiac Catheterization – 2402	25.00	48.00	2249.00	50260.00	1.11%	0.10%
Radiology – 2500	110.00	2118.00	2249.00	50250.00	4.89%	4.21%
CT Scan – 2501	38.00	246.00	303.00	7119.00	12.54%	3.46%
Ultrasound – 2502	5.00	98.00	80.00	2057.00	6.25%	4.76%
MRI – 2503	15.00	291.00	323.00	7883.00	4.64%	3.69%
Pharmacy – 2600	4.00	283.00	1280.00	30911.00	0.31%	0.92%
Nuclear Medicine – 2700	19.00	457.00	462.00	11789.00	4.11%	3.88%
Laboratory—Central – 2800	210.00	3501.00	4567.00	92456.00	4.60%	3.79%
Laboratory—Satellites – 2801	22.00	267.00	423.00	8743.00	5.20%	3.05%
Materials Management – 3000	1.00	84.00	487.00	7826.00	0.21%	1.07%

(continued on following page)

TABLE 2.2 *(continued)*

Department						
Materials Distribution – 3001	19.00	89.00	257.00	6954.00	7.39%	1.28%
Central Supply – 3002	46.00	1598.00	1448.00	32407.00	3.18%	4.93%
Facilities Management – 3100	3.00	11.00	211.00	2371.00	1.42%	0.46%
Plant Operations – 3101	36.00	737.00	639.00	14579.00	5.63%	5.06%
Maintenance Operations – 3102	54.00	853.00	572.00	11961.00	9.44%	7.13%
Biomedical Engineering – 3103	3.00	144.00	183.00	4653.00	1.64%	3.09%
Environmental Services – 3200	189.00	5073.00	3813.00	83972.00	4.96%	6.04%
Laundry and Linen – 3201	3.00	289.00	219.00	4678.00	1.37%	6.18%
Food Services – 3300	31.00	1158.00	2166.00	53854.00	1.43%	2.15%
Cafeteria – 3301	39.00	39.00	588.00	868.00	6.63%	4.49%
Dieticians – 3302	12.00	433.00	867.00	19019.00	1.38%	2.28%
Safety and Security – 3400	13.00	469.00	493.00	12304.00	2.64%	3.81%
Central Transportation – 3500	22.00	22.00	840.00	474.00	2.62%	4.64%
Telecommunications – 3600	13.00	334.00	733.00	18005.00	1.77%	1.86%
Information Services – 4000	95.00	2459.00	1796.00	40901.00	5.29%	6.01%
Health Information Management – 4100	89.00	2501.00	1903.00	38932.00	4.68%	6.42%
Transcription – 4101	30.00	786.00	910.00	9987.00	3.30%	7.87%
Tumor Registry – 4102	0.00	43.00	80.00	1883.00	0.00%	2.28%
Executive Administration – 4300	0.00	32.00	780.00	17890.00	0.00%	0.18%
Finance Administration – 4400	0.00	20.00	320.00	7654.00	0.00%	0.26%
General Accounting – 4500	2.00	34.00	480.00	11870.00	0.42%	0.29%
Patient Registration – 4600	87.00	4780.00	1568.00	87638.00	5.55%	5.45%
Patient Accounting – 4700	98.00	5432.00	1879.00	92430.00	5.22%	5.88%
Total	2172.00	60360.00	65608.00	1525255.00	3.31%	3.96%

Issued 11/25/04

in the first place. The title of Report 1 indicates that it is for Overtime Hours Worked by Pay Period and YTD. The recipient(s) may be the leadership group—CEO, COO, CFO, vice president of operations, or vice president of nursing. The purpose is to create a summary, by department, of the overtime hours worked for a given period versus the total overtime hours worked to date, and knowing this information presumably allows the senior administrators to understand the overtime hours being used.

However, Report 1 does not yield any use for the reader. It has six columns of data, all of which are "actual" hours worked. Because of this, the report is not inclusive and does not allow for comparisons against a variety of other data. In this case, the two most important pieces of information missing are budget (or goal) and volume. Without the ability to make such a comparison, the readers cannot work toward achieving their purpose.

Furthermore, the design of Report 1 is neither understandable nor straightforward. Here are seven bad elements:

1. Title includes the abbreviation YTD. Abbreviations should never be used in reports, because such use is an assumption that every reader knows what the abbreviation stands for. YTD should be spelled out to Year to Date.
2. Title and column headings are in all caps. Only the first letter of each word should be capitalized for readability.
3. Numbers in each column include decimal points, even though the two digits afterward are all zeros. This does nothing but further clutter the report.
4. No commas are used to indicate that some numbers are in thousands.
5. Rows are sorted by cost center number in descending order, but these numbers are the second grouping of data on each line, not the first.
6. Rows are not initially sorted by department. (More about proper sorting in a later discussion.)
7. Data in each column are centered. Numbers should be left justified to enhance readability.

While Report 1 is presumably accurate, it is not timely. A look at the small type at the bottom of the table indicates that the report was issued ten days after the pay period ended (11/25/04 versus 11/15/04). Reports are more actionable when they are current.

Reports can only be cost effective if the cost to create them is outweighed by the benefits they provide to the readers. Because of all the problems in Report 1, no benefit is presented, and it therefore fails the cost-effectiveness test.

Report 1 also does not include any commentary from the report developer. Such a narrative addresses the issues identified in the report. Lack of a commentary may be a result of the inability of the developer to identify problem issues because of the report's poor design, or it may be because the developer does not know that he or she has the responsibility to provide a narrative discussing the issues.

How to Improve Report 1

There are many ways to improve Report 1 to meet the ten elements of good reporting.

First, the seven items of poor design mentioned earlier should be fixed:

1. Do not use abbreviations.
2. Capitalize only the first letter of each word to allow the reader's eye to recognize and better understand the column headers.
3. Get rid of all the digits after the decimal, as they add no further information to the analysis.
4. Add commas to separate the thousands.
5. Resort the rows from highest to lowest variance.
6. Resort the rows by department.
7. Left justify all the column headers and rows to improve readability.

Second, address the most important element—the content. Ask what Report 1 is trying to achieve (the purpose). In this case, the leadership group is trying to determine which departments are violating Pleasant Flats's overtime policy. The current report does not give this information because it only includes actual data. Therefore, budget and/or goal information as well as volume information need to be added to enable the readers to compare the extra hours used with the extra hours worked.

A good report includes volume, budget, and actual data that become the basis for actionable, information-driven outcomes. Therefore, Report 1 should include hours per unit of service information, arrayed from the highest to the lowest variance. Table 2.3 represents the ideal report that could have and should have been created so that the leadership group could foster accountability in the medical center. This report consists of only 26 lines, rather than 3 pages, featuring the departments that did not meet their overtime goals for the given pay period on a year-to-date basis. It has only 26 lines, and yet this report is so much more actionable than Report 1 presented to the leadership. Although this ideal report took more work, the hard work really occurs only once. Once the proper elements and design have been determined and established in the beginning, the report can run independently.

What matters is not the degree of difficulty of producing a report but the outcomes the report yields—that is, did the report achieve its desired result, which is to give the decision maker the right information?

Sample Report 2

Another very ugly report is presented in Figure 2.5 (page 40). Report 2 is an actual report, developed by a hospital finance department and used at the senior management level. This report has a number of problems, but perhaps the greatest one is its lack of simplicity. In other words, Report 2 is too complicated; therefore, its information is not accessible to the reader. What is this report trying to accomplish anyway? It appears that its creator was attempting to represent the operating margin in a variety of ways. In doing so, the report shows month- and year-to-date dollars as well as what appears to be year-to-date operating margin percentage (Ytd Om rg/Orev). Because of its complexity, Report 2 fails in displaying the information needed to achieve the goal.

Here are some of this report's specific problems:

1. Lines that go up and lines that go sideways are all over the chart.
2. Columns are used, but it is unclear how they relate to the lines.
3. Numbers are used at every data point, cluttering up the chart.

The Power of Clinical and Financial Metrics

TABLE 2.3 PLEASANT FLATS MEDICAL CENTER'S OVERTIME HOURS WORKED PER VOLUME, BY PAY PERIOD AND YEAR-TO-DATE, PAY PERIOD 24 (11/02–11/15/2004)

	Overtime Hours per Volume Pay Period 24			Overtime Hours per Volume Year-to-Date Pay Period 24		
	Actual	*Budget*	*% Variance*	*Actual*	*Budget*	*% Variance*
Biomedical engineering – 3103	0.13	0.09	53.6	0.27	0.19	44.8
Laboratory—satellites – 2801	0.99	0.69	42.1	0.51	0.38	35.4
Nursing float – 102	0.00	0.09	100.0	0.02	0.01	30.7
Environmental services – 3200	8.40	8.68	3.2	9.59	7.52	27.5
Surgery – 1500	9.88	6.18	59.9	8.43	6.62	27.5
3 Southwest – 1112	9.62	5.25	83.2	17.24	13.56	27.1
Health information management – 4100	3.96	3.47	13.9	4.73	3.76	25.7
3 Northeast – 1113	6.82	7.50	9.1	24.23	19.57	23.8
Information services – 4000	4.22	4.34	2.7	4.65	3.76	23.6
Food services – 3300	0.55	0.52	6.9	0.98	0.80	22.8
Home health services – 1800	2.22	1.82	22.2	4.64	3.83	21.0
Laboratory—central – 2800	3.82	3.53	8.5	2.90	2.41	–20.1

Department					
Day treatment – 1402	0.00	1.98	100.0	0.38	0.33	16.1
Cardiac Catheterization – 2402	104.17	85.71	21.5	8.00	7.14	12.0
Telecommunications – 3600	0.58	0.43	33.1	0.63	0.56	12.0
Patient accounting – 4700	4.36	3.73	16.7	10.27	9.26	11.0
Hospice – 1801	17.39	12.00	44.9	9.49	8.67	9.5
Case management – 103	0.7	1.04	27.5	0.09	0.08	9.3
Nuclear medicine – 2700	25.00	30.00	16.7	26.14	23.96	9.1
Post-acute care unit – 1501	4.94	4.71	4.9	6.41	5.88	9.0
Cardiology – 2400	5.69	6.15	7.5	6.28	5.83	7.7
Maintenance operations – 3102	2.40	2.43	1.3	1.61	1.50	7.2
Plant operations – 3101	1.60	1.35	18.9	1.39	1.32	5.9
Inpatient psychiatric – 1400	42.86	47.57	9.9	20.63	20.02	3.0
Labor and delivery – 1200	83.57	75.00	11.4	118.96	115.63	2.9
Lactation – 2101	8.16	11.54	29.3	4.20	4.17	0.8

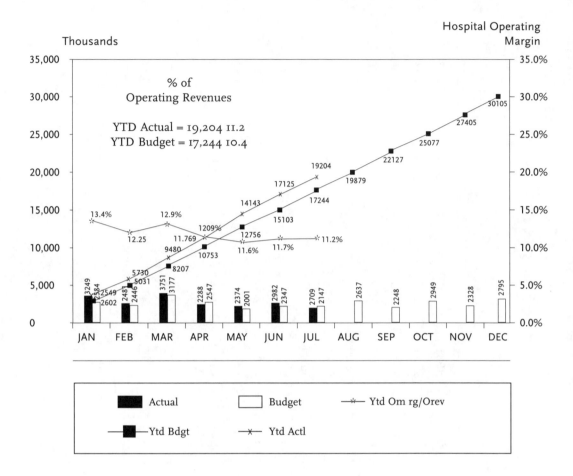

FIGURE 2.5 ANYTOWN MEDICAL CENTER'S HOSPITAL OPERATING MARGIN, FOR THE MONTH AND YEAR TO DATE JULY 2004

4. Numbers sit in the middle of the chart, adding to the clutter.
5. There are two sets of Y axes, making the reader unsure which data belong on which axes.
6. Different font types are used, leading to the sense of ugliness.
7. A legend is provided, but it uses abbreviations without explanation, such as "YTD Actl," "YTD Bdgt" and "Ytd Om rg/Orev."

Report 2 is awful. Its creator was trying to cram three reports into one, which is a common problem in report design. This should not be done.

Some improvements that can be made to this report include the following:

1. Break up the components into more manageable, multiple charts.
2. Whenever possible, do not use more than one Y axis.
3. Use one font type for consistency.
4. Limit the data points so that the reader's eye can concentrate on the important elements.
5. Do not use abbreviations in the legend. Again, using abbreviations assumes that the reader understands them, which is not always the case.

Overall, when designing reports, keep in mind that, in most cases, less is more. Step into the shoes of the reader to visualize what component of a report is most important to their decisions. Then, present that information in a simple and appealing manner.

The Good: Sample Reports 3 and 4

Ugly and bad reports are easy to pick on, as so many of them exist and come in different varieties. It is still a challenge for many organizations to produce reports that are easy to look at, understandable at a glance, and actionable by the recipient. Two examples of good reports are illustrated in the next pages; they can be adopted by any organization. Report 3 is common and is easy to produce and disseminate. Report 4 embodies all ten elements of good design, enabling its reader to see its point and to generate a decision.

Figure 2.6 is an example of a report that is elegantly presented and includes information that indicates, in summary, the financial results of the organization over the past month. It meets all ten elements of good design, revealing important figures that the organization expects to achieve. It is simple and clear, stating relevant, useful, and comprehensive facts that are not only accurate and up-to-date but also can be used for comparison. Most importantly, at the right side of the report is a short narrative that enhances the reader's understanding of the figures.

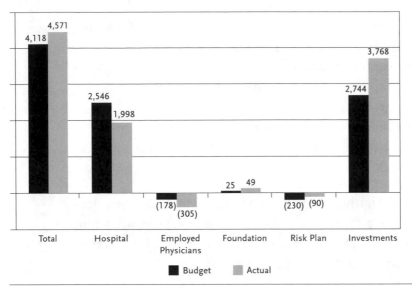

FIGURE 2.6 NET INCOME BY DIVISION, DECEMBER 2004 (THOUSANDS OMMITTED)

■ Budget   ▨ Actual

Report 4 is presented in Figure 2.7. Although it is certainly more complex than Report 3, it is able to convey, in its design, a story that can lead to action. In this case, the report recipient is the hospital president, who was unsatisfied with the level of the organization's accounts receivable. The president requested a report that indicates the reasons cash was not being received by the hospital in a timely and reliable way. The report developer reviewed a variety of available data and prepared a report showing the impact of the patients who had been discharged but whose bills had not yet been produced and sent to the responsible payer.

The results of Report 4, across an 18-month trend period, were startling. As is quite evident in the report, the dramatic increase in the discharged and not final billed (DNFB) in both the inpatient and outpatient categories was the single greatest cause of a slowdown in bills production. Although the hospital CFO was responsible for reporting the entire accounts receivable activities to the board, she did not have authority for the coding function, which is the last step before producing the bills. This was the primary reason for the high DNFB rate.

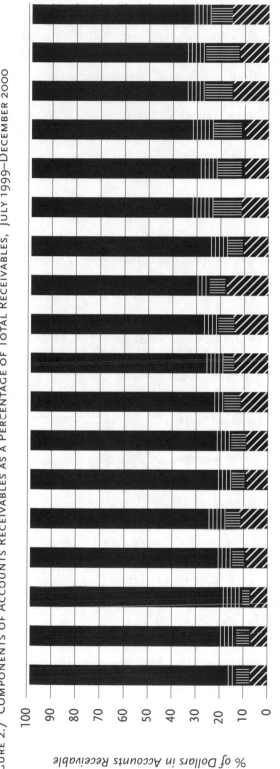

FIGURE 2.7 COMPONENTS OF ACCOUNTS RECEIVABLES AS A PERCENTAGE OF TOTAL RECEIVABLES, JULY 1999–DECEMBER 2000

% of Dollars in Accounts Receivable

	Jul-99	Aug-99	Sep-99	Oct-99	Nov-99	Dec-99	Jan-00	Feb-00	Mar-00	Apr-00	May-00	Jun-00	Jul-00	Aug-00	Sep-00	Oct-00	Nov-00	Dec-00
Billed A/R	31,711	33,288	35,556	34,882	32,661	33,040	30,688	28,927	30,089	30,396	27,518	26,587	25,184	27,619	26,852	25,610	24,707	25,799
In-house	1,793	3,326	3,683	3,254	3,447	2,672	2,746	2,185	2,261	2,798	2,352	2,360	3,149	3,032	3,865	3,333	2,939	2,217
DNFB O/P	2,073	2,058	1,416	1,999	2,305	1,895	2,106	2,383	2,226	2,739	2,542	2,328	4,923	4,515	4,993	5,327	5,894	4,510
DNFB I/P	2,665	2,975	2,974	4,208	5,262	3,935	3,651	4,171	5,488	5,726	6,677	3,506	3,973	3,977	4,007	5,534	4,539	5,232

This chart indicates that the discharged and not final billed categories (DNFB), both inpatient (I/P) and outpatient (O/P), have been the cause of the greatest increases in the accounts receivable (A/R). In July of 1999, these two categories made up about 12 percent of the outstanding receivables ($4.7 million). In December of 2000, these same two categories made up about 26 percent of the receivables ($9.7 million).

Report 4 does contain a narrative commentary at the bottom, but its creator refrained from making this most obvious observation knowing that the reader (hospital president) was aware of the fact that the CFO had no authority over coding. In this case, it worked! The president looked at the graph for 60 seconds, and then issued an order that hence forth the coding department would report to the CFO, which was an instantaneous and binding decision. The trending in the graph produced information that would have been ineffective in a verbal commentary. The picture represented by the graph was irrefutable.

Most reports can have this kind of outcome if they are created to maximize impact rather than to merely list or rehash data. When the results of the report are given more emphasis than the process of reporting, the reports, containing metrics of all dimensions, take on new meaning. Any report creator can achieve this type of success by changing his or her reporting direction.

The Bad and the Ugly Versus the Good: Sample of a Physician Report

In this discussion of reporting hospital information, it is imperative that some space is given to physician reporting. Table 2.4 contains data that represent some sort of outcomes. At first glance, however, what outcomes are represented in this report is unclear. At a closer reading (by someone who understands the language of such reports), this report shows average charges (Avg Tot \$/H_ac) by physician (Last Att #), within diagnosis-related group (DRG), and the total number of cases performed by the physicians within a time period (# Pts/H_ac).

This report is essentially unreadable, particularly because the column headers are so cryptic with all sorts of abbreviation. Even when the headers are recognizable, the reader is still unable to make a decision based on the array of the data included.

Figure 2.8 provides a much better way to show the same data, displaying the principles of good design that lead to useful information for decision making. This report graphs the current-year data along with the previous-year data. In doing so, a trending is created, adding information to the analysis. As in Table 2.4, this graph in Figure 2.8 shows the physicians' charges and cases, but it arrays these numbers in a way that highlights which physicians are using more resources

TABLE 2.4 GROUP FILTER: DRG IS EQUAL TO 127 88 132 89 182 391 373 121 296 138 390 183 15 79 143 209 96 14 122 141 174 90

DISCHARGE DATE: 07/01/2003–04/30/2004

DRG	DRG ADesc	Last Att #	Avg Tot $ /H_ac	# Pts /H_ac
14	CerebrovDxexTIA	000120	10836	4
14	CerebrovDxexTIA	000104	8378	2
14	CerebrovDxexTIA	000114	5586	6
14	CerebrovDxexTIA	000103	5161	2
14	CerebrovDxexTIA	000110	4877	2
14	CerebrovDxexTIA	001198	4850	1
14	CerebrovDxexTIA	000124	4704	4
14	CerebrovDxexTIA	000115	4346	4
15	TIA&PrecerbOccl	000104	6595	1
15	TIA&PrecerbOccl	000120	6192	4
15	TIA&PrecerbOccl	000115	5992	7
15	TIA&PrecerbOccl	001199	5977	2
15	TIA&PrecerbOccl	000339	5935	1
15	TIA&PrecerbOccl	000103	5433	2
15	TIA&PrecerbOccl	000114	4897	3
15	TIA&PrecerbOccl	001198	4684	2
15	TIA&PrecerbOccl	000112	3497	4
15	TIA&PrecerbOccl	000110	3390	2
79	Resp Inf > 17wCC	000110	11458	5
79	Resp Inf > 17wCC	000112	9397	4
79	Resp Inf > 17wCC	000120	8066	7
79	Resp Inf > 17wCC	000115	7323	1
79	Resp Inf > 17wCC	000124	5592	11
88	COPD	000112	7921	2
88	COPD	000104	7041	9
88	COPD	001189	6183	1
88	COPD	000102	5599	1
88	COPD	001199	5191	4
88	COPD	000120	5039	5
88	COPD	000339	4795	1
88	COPD	000114	4589	15
88	COPD	000110	4518	9
88	COPD	000115	4159	6
88	COPD	000103	4060	3
88	COPD	000124	3849	44

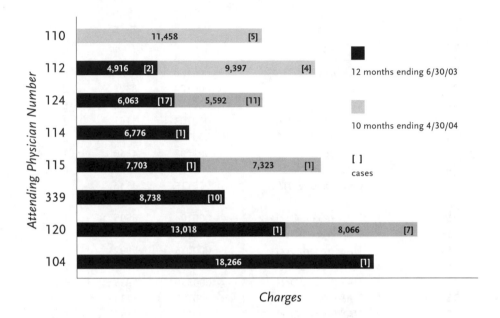

Charges

This chart indicates that Attending Physician 124, who has the greatest number of DRG 79 cases in both the 12 months ending June 30, 2003 and the 10 months ending April 30, 2004, also has the lowest charges (and presumably lowest costs). This is advantageous to the hospital. The organization should establish a multidisciplinary team consisting of physicians and other clinical and financial management and staff to discuss how to reduce resource consumption.

and which are using less across time. It has a clean look, and the reader can quickly distinguish the results of the various physicians.

Most interestingly, Figure 2.8 includes a narrative—one of the elements of good reporting. The narrative not only explains the results given but also states a direction based on the findings, although some may find the last line of this narrative unacceptable, believing that the report creator (who is perhaps a financial or clinical analyst) should not be directing the reader to a conclusion. However, without this direction, the narrative is not as effective. While the report recipient has every right to disagree with the analyst's conclusion, at the time the report is created nobody has a better understanding of the data and information than the person who just assembled that information—that is, the creator. Thus, preparing reports and rendering strong conclusions can make reports much more informative.

Jane's head was spinning. So much improvement was available to Pleasant Flats. These opportunities existed, but Jane needed to sort them out in an actionable and effective way.

Having interviewed the board chair as well as some of the members of the finance committee, Jane learned that they never read beyond page 3 of the 30-page monthly report and 25 of these pages were never reviewed by the powers that be. Jane took this as a mandate for change. Having learned quite a bit about the elements of good reporting, including how to design a good report and how to avoid the bad and ugly ones, Jane set out to remake the board reporting package. Her first goal was to reduce it.

In the end, the board package was reduced from 30 pages of unused data to 10 pages of understandable information. She started with a ratio analysis report (or key success factors), followed by a narrative explaining the significant variances from the budgeted goals. Many of these explanations came from the managers' electronically generated responses to the alerts they received immediately after their reporting system uploaded the information. Thus, Jane and her staff were able to prepare more effective reports in a timely manner.

Jane also automated much of the financial and clinical reporting through the use of a balanced scorecard. This allowed senior leadership and the board to quickly evaluate those indicators that had been selected as most important to Pleasant Flats's success.

The board was very pleased. By getting less data and more information, the board members realized that they had been missing good analysis in the previous years. The improved package made them fully appreciate the information they were now receiving. As for Jane, she had secured her tenure at the medical center for years to come.

PRACTICAL TIPS

☛ Make every report actionable. If no action can be taken based on findings from a report, do not create the report or do not have it done.

☛ When reducing overly long board packages, consider putting the most important information—such as a ratio analysis/key success factors report—on page 1. It summarizes all the important elements of the balance sheet and the statement of operations in a format that is comparable and able to be benchmarked.

☛ Adopt all ten elements of good reporting into every report generated by the organization.

CHAPTER THREE

Adopting Benchmarking and Best Practices to Achieve Superior Results

Sam Barnes woke up in a cold sweat, pain radiating from several parts of his body. He didn't know what was going on, but whatever it was, it was pain that wouldn't go away. Relentless. Unnerving. Frightening.

He didn't know what to do. Should he call his primary physician for some advice? What would his physician say at 3 o'clock in the morning anyway? Probably for him to go to the nearest emergency room (ER). Sam thought about cutting out a step and just going. After all, the ER should be staffed to take care of whatever the problem was, but he was a little bit apprehensive. How good were the local hospital's ER, physicians, and nurses? Sam knew that it was a growing community hospital, but he was not sure about its technological capabilities or its ability to diagnose his pain. He read in the newspaper that Pleasant Flats Medical Center was just completing a $90 million expansion and renovation, part of which involved the ER. This was probably a good sign, he thought. Still, he had never seen any independent assessments or evaluations of the hospital, not in the newspapers or magazines, nor had he heard any particular word of mouth about its ER.

What Sam wanted was competency. He was not concerned about how exceptionally good the hospital was; he just wanted to be sure that they could diagnose and treat him in an efficient and professional manner. He did not feel the need to find "the best," typically denoted by the big downtown academic medical centers.

How could he judge the competency of this hospital? Right now, he needed help and was going to the closest facility. He had little or no choice at this point because, like most Americans, he had not done research on this before he needed to know it. All he could do was hope that the hospital's administration had adopted practices that would improve his chances of being treated in the most appropriate, efficient, and effective manner. He hoped that the hospital used practices and techniques that had proved successful at other medical centers.

WHAT DOES IT really mean to be the best—to have established the best practice in your particular industry, your particular talent, your particular skill? It is very possible to achieve the lofty heights representing the best practices. Very possible, but it is not easy, takes a lot of hard work, and involves following a number of roadmaps.

Over the past few decades, the concept of best practices has sprung up within all industries. This idea certainly has not been confined to the United States alone but has become commonplace throughout the world. This chapter provides a window into the world of hospital best practices, discussing definitions, history, and examples of benchmarking. A case study featuring a particular best-practice health system is also presented.

DEFINITIONS

Best practices can be defined as policies, procedures, methods, and systems that enable administrators, through research and comparison, to achieve superior results in several leadership and management categories. Comparisons in the following four primary categories can be made using hundreds of metric indicators:

- Customer satisfaction
- Quality indicators
- Clinical outcomes
- Financial results

Benchmarking is the process of comparing practices and services in your own organization with those of peer organizations within the industry. *Benchmarks* are standards of excellence and achievement against which similar things may be measured or judged. As these measurements are interpreted against your own organization, it becomes easier to determine which companies are performing in the best manner. It is from these best performers that best practices can be studied and adopted.

In his autobiography, the founder of Wal-Mart, Sam Walton (1992) quotes one of his most experienced and long-time managers Charlie Cade, who was reminiscing about working with Walton in the early 1960s: "I remember [Sam] saying over and over again, 'Go in and check out the competition. Check everyone who is our competition. And don't look for the bad. Look for the good. If you get one good idea, that's one more than you went into the store with, and we must try to incorporate it into our company. We are not really concerned with what they're doing wrong, we're concerned with what they're doing right, and everyone is doing something right'."

No better description of adopting best practices as a management credo can top this Walton passage. As we all know, Wal-Mart went on to become the world's largest retailer, in part because the company relentlessly determined best practices throughout its industry and adopted/adapted to these practices throughout the organization. This same opportunity is available in the healthcare industry. To access this opportunity, however, organizations must adopt benchmarking as an ongoing, coordinated management technique.

Benchmarking allows the benchmarked organization to gain a different, and often better, perspective on its own situation. It allows the organization to think outside the box while gaining awareness to what similar organizations are doing. Learning about outcomes achieved by its peers enables the organization to make decisions. For example, it can compare its metric outcomes to its peers and determine (1) the reasons that it is achieving different results (better or worse) and (2) the changes it needs to make to improve or maintain its results.

In essence, benchmarking is a tool for improving performance in that it requires an organization to examine others' practices that have led to best results. The process of benchmarking and applying lessons learned involves four basic steps:

1. Know in detail your own processes.
2. Analyze the processes of others.
3. Compare your own performance with that of others analyzed.
4. Implement the steps necessary to close the performance gap.

HISTORY

Benchmarking has a long and proud history in industries outside of healthcare. It has been used to make consistent and long-term improvements to inputs and outcomes. Just think about the automobile industry, for example. As it was riding high in the 1960s, the Japanese automakers were scrutinizing every aspect of the U.S. automakers' production, scanning for the best- and worst-employed practices. In doing so, the Japanese were redeveloping their own industry, intent on surpassing the Americans in design, production, cost management, and productivity.

The Japanese went around the world touring and benchmarking all the best organizations—a practice they termed "industry tours." Their focus was on others' processes instead of products, and they used steps that are the same as benchmarking:

1. Research published data to define the best.
2. Contact the best, and schedule a visit.
3. Visit the best, and carefully select pertinent data.
4. Return home, and adopt (or adapt) the lessons learned in your own organization to gain a competitive advantage.

As a result, Japanese carmakers achieved significant breakthroughs that allowed them to improve their market share while substantially cutting their costs. The upshot of this one-way benchmarking is that when the American automakers saw the changes being wrought by the new Japanese techniques, benchmarking and best-practice analysis led the Americans to adopt many of the practices developed by the Japanese.

In the 1960s, IBM began to use internal benchmarking activities. IBM gained a significant international competitive advantage through determining the best production processes internally and adopting them as the corporate standard. In the 1970s, Xerox decided to follow IBM's example by comparing its U.S. products with those of its Japanese affiliate Fuji-Xerox. The initial benchmarking program was so successful that management later incorporated it as a fundamental element in Xerox's worldwide improvement efforts. This improvement process was so pronounced that Xerox is often credited as being the forerunner of the benchmarking movement.

Some of the major multinational corporations that have used benchmarking to achieve breakthrough success include the following (Harrington and Harrington 1996):

- Kodak
- Digital Equipment
- Xerox
- 3M
- AT&T
- Boeing
- DuPont
- Hewlett Packard
- Johnson & Johnson

In the healthcare industry, and particularly hospitals, numerous benchmarking opportunities are available. Several major proprietary benchmarking organizations provide a variety of services to their customers. Chief among these services is the generation of quarterly reports of the client's actual financial and clinical results compared with different peer groupings. Such information allows the hospital to determine its standing among other facilities. These reports are very valuable for any information-driven hospital. If used properly, these reports can drive improvements.

Interestingly, benchmarking is not always embraced by all members of a hospital's management and senior leadership. These members either do not like their organization compared to others (particularly when the results are unfavorable) or do not believe that the benchmarking outcomes are valid or relevant. Part of this attitude stems from bad history in healthcare industry benchmarking in the 1970s and early 1980s, when inaccurate results were yielded because of a lack of reasonable comparability provided by the primary benchmarking services of that time. Bad history is hard to overcome, but it is necessary to put this past to rest and move forward. The big proprietary benchmark-service providers today have done a remarkable job of ensuring reasonable comparability and providing value-added information.

BEST PRACTICES IN THE HEALTHCARE INDUSTRY

In this discussion of best-practice performers within healthcare, the generally accepted criteria for best practices have to be addressed. Figure 3.1 is a partial list of companies that provide best-practice information. Each of these benchmarking-service providers has developed its own definition, standard, and justification for selecting a best-practice organization.

There is never just one, all-encompassing answer to who or what is the "best." However, to determine whether a particular hospital or health system rose up to the standard of superior performance, two highly regarded services were reviewed—Solucient's 100 Top Hospitals® and the Malcolm Baldrige National Quality Award. The 100 Top Hospitals® survey has great credibility within the healthcare industry, and the Baldrige award has great recognition and credibility in all industries. Best performers selected by each service have achieved results that are measurable, verifiable, and sustainable.

Solucient's 100 Top Hospitals®: National Benchmarks for Success

The 100 Top Hospitals® is a program that measures hospitals' (small, medium, large, and teaching organizations) level of performance in various categories. Organizations that perform at the highest levels are then selected and included in a publication aimed to not only applaud the efforts of these hospitals but also to inform others of the benchmarks attained.

The publication has evolved into being the first national comparative balanced scorecard that covers an entire segment of the healthcare industry. Its content validity and utility to boards of trustees and healthcare executives are demonstrated in a research article by University of

Michigan professors John Griffith and Jeffrey Alexander (2002). Produced by the Center for Healthcare Improvement, a division of Solucient, Inc., the 100 Top Hospitals® program was initiated in 1993 to do the following:

- Identify superior management teams using solely objective statistical methods that are open to scrutiny via use of public data sources (i.e., Medicare Cost Report and MedPAR billing files).
- Identify hospitals that are consistent top performers, using a comparative balanced scorecard approach to measure quality of care, efficiency of operations, financial performance, and positive response from customers.
- Build a national hospital-benchmark database that reflects current and long-term governance and managerial performance.

Program Criteria

To ensure fair judging of the best organizationwide performance, Solucient annually reviews the program criteria and implements improvements. The 2003 edition (published in 2004) includes nine separate criteria or metrics. According to Solucient, these criteria form a balanced-scorecard-type matrix that, if used at a high level, will ensure that the hospital achieves high-quality clinical (product quality) results, financial strength, efficient operations, and positive customer response (growth of business). The nine criteria are listed in Table 3.1.

Each of these criteria is a metric that has specific applicability to a hospital's business and is actionable by management. The product quality indicators represent the gross clinical outcomes in terms of expected mortality and complications of the inpatient population. The financial indicators signify levels of profitability, ability to support debt incurred, and soundness of long-term investment. The efficiency indicators denote the organization's ability to control its (1) operational efficiency in terms of expense per adjusted discharge and (2) clinical efficiency in terms of its adjusted length of stay. Customer response is currently measured by the percentage growth in the community that the hospital serves. The final criterion—coding specificity rate—is not a measure of overall organizational performance, but it is actionable by management. This metric attempts to address the value that manage-

TABLE 3.1 SOLUCIENT'S 100 TOP HOSPITALS® CRITERIA, 2003

Indicators	Calculations
Quality	
Risk-adjusted mortality	The number of actual deaths divided by the number expected, given the risk of death for each patient; based on Solucient's statistical modeling
Risk-adjusted complications	The number of actual complications divided by the number expected, given the risk of death for each patient; based on Solucient's expected complications rate index model
Operating Efficiency and Financial Health	
Profitability (operating profit margin)	The difference between total operating revenue and total operating expense, expressed as a percentage of total operating revenues
Expense per adjusted discharge	The total operating expenses divided by the number of adjusted discharges case mix and wage adjusted
Cash flow to total debt	The sum of net income, current depreciation expense, and interest expense divided by total liabilities
Tangible assets per adjusted discharge	Total property, plant, and equipment at a hospital less accumulated depreciation divided by the total number of adjusted acute care discharges at the facility
Severity-adjusted average length of stay	The average patient length of stay, adjusted for differences in severity of illness
Responsiveness to the Community	
Growth in percentage of community served	The hospital's one-year growth in percentage of patients served by the hospital (expressed as a percentage); each year's percentage of patients served is calculated as the number of Medicare patients discharged by the hospital divided by the number of Medicare patients discharged by hospitals in the same "referral" region in Solucient's study sampling frame
Coding specificity rate	The number of patient records that are "specific" divided by the total number of patient records; Solucient is valuing coding that is more specific and less "not otherwise specified"

Source: Used with permission from Solucient, LLC.

ment places on the accuracy of its decision support information. As metrics, all of these indicators represent opportunities gained or lost.

By themselves, the numerical outcomes are relatively meaningless. However, compared to the results achieved in the last several years, these numbers allow a hospital to determine a positive or negative trend in each key managerial area and point to the development and progress needed toward an organizationwide culture of performance improvement. Further, when compared against nationwide peer organizations, the indicators take on full meaning. Each hospital that reviews its own data against those of its peers can now determine how well it is performing relative to others. The national comparisons also demonstrate how well the hospital is likely to function under pay-for-performance schemes, given that pay for performance is based on the ability of a hospital to outperform its peers on an ongoing basis. This information also allows any hospital to move toward best-practice performance, should it so choose.

To achieve greater validity in the outcomes, the program segregates more than 3,000 U.S. hospitals into five peer groups. In 2003, these peer groups were represented as shown in Table 3.2.

What Do the 100 Top Hospitals Do Differently?

As the results suggest, the 100 Top Hospitals achieve outcomes that far exceed those of their peers. William M. Mercer consultants conducted research in 1996 to identify common management characteristics of executive teams in hospitals that had been selected by the 100 Top Hospitals program three or more times. In most cases, the researchers found these management teams to have the following:

- Superior communication: few, if any, barriers to the information flow in any direction existed.
- Clarity of goals: growth and continuous performance improvement were the focus.
- Emphasis on quality improvement and cost reduction: these were considered in improvement discussions and in goal setting.
- Well-designed infrastructure to support goal achievement and performance monitoring: this was achieved through consistent reporting of the metric goals to enhance decision making.

TABLE 3.2 100 TOP HOSPITAL PEER GROUPS, 2003

Peer Groups	Number of Benchmark Hospitals	Total Number of Facilities
Small hospitals (25–99 beds)	20	1,226
Medium hospitals (100–249 beds)	20	1,072
Large community hospitals (250+ beds)	20	280
Teaching hospitals (200+ beds and sponsorship of at least 3 graduate medical education programs overall or an intern-to-resident per bed ratio of at least 1 to 3.3)	25	376
Major teaching hospitals (400+ beds and at least 10 graduate medical education programs overall or an intern-to-resident per bed ratio of at least 1 to 4)	15	141

Source: Used with permission from Solucient, LLC.

- Team value: there was alignment vertically and horizontally and a minimum of infighting.

Over the past 11 years, Solucient has reported additional findings, based on the use of different metrics and databases, about differences between consistent award winners and nonwinners. The winning hospitals do the following:

- Treat sicker patients, yet save more lives: this is based on case mix index and survival rates.
- Perform more efficiently, yet have lower costs: this is based on faster return to daily life and expense per adjusted discharge.
- Treat significantly more patients: this is based on admission per bed.
- Have fewer staff, yet ensure equal employee pay: this is based on full time equivalents (FTEs) per adjusted discharges and five-year salary and benefits per FTE trends.

- Serve a larger percentage of their community.
- Use new technology in a more strategic manner.
- Employ better business practices.
- Have more community outreach programs.
- Have superior clinical practice outcomes.

In summary, 100 Top Hospital winners are considered best across various metric indicators that have proven reliable in measuring success in hospital operations. Recognizing the metrics and moving any hospital organization toward higher value are likely to push any organization to improved performance.

Malcolm Baldrige National Quality Award

Named after the 26th secretary of the U.S. Department of Commerce, the Malcolm Baldrige National Quality Award (MBNQA) was established by Congress in 1987 to enhance the competitiveness of U.S. organizations. The award may be presented to five types of organizations—manufacturers, service companies, small businesses, educational organizations, and healthcare organizations—but it is not given for specific products or services. Between 1988 and 2004, 62 Baldrige Awards were presented to 59 organizations.

The award is given to organizations that show exemplary achievements in seven areas:

1. Leadership
2. Strategic planning
3. Focus on patients, other customers, and markets
4. Measurement, analysis, and knowledge management
5. Focus on staff
6. Process management
7. Organizational performance results

All applicants for the Baldrige Award undergo a rigorous examination process that involves a minimum of 300 hours of review by an independent board of examiners, who are primarily from the private sector. Final-stage applicants receive about 1,000 hours of review and are visited by teams of examiners to clarify questions and verify information. Each applicant receives a report that cites its strengths and opportunities for improvement.

More information on the award and winners, including Baptist Hospital in Pensacola, Florida (which won in 2003); St. Luke's Hospital in Kansas City, Missouri (which won in 2003); and Robert Wood Johnson University Hospital in Hamilton, New Jersey (which won in 2004), is available online at www.quality.nist.gov.

Program Criteria

The Baldrige Award is designed to promote excellence in organizational performance, recognizes the quality and performance achievements of organizations, and publicizes successful performance strategies. It uses metrics-based criteria to determine the level at which the candidate organization is performing. Figure 3.2 lists the 1,000 points by which candidates are judged. Baldrige reviewers evaluate the organizations against strict criteria to determine their worthiness for the award.

The Baldrige program guide (Baldrige National Quality Program 2004a) recommends the following ten-step assessment and action plan to any organization interested in moving toward the Baldrige status:

1. Identify the boundaries of the organization to be assessed.
2. Select seven champions—one for each of the seven Baldrige categories.
3. Decide on the format for and scope of the self-assessment and action plan.
4. Senior leaders and champions should prepare the organizational profile.
5. Practice self-assessment techniques with the champions, using Item 1.1 (see Figure 3.2).
6. Champions should select category teams. Champions and teams should prepare a response for their assigned items.
7. Share responses among teams, and finalize the findings. Identify key strengths and gaps in category responses.
8. Prioritize the organization's key strengths and opportunities for improvement.
9. Develop and implement an action plan for improvement.
10. Evaluate and improve the self-assessment and action processes.

1. *Leadership*
    1.1 Organizational leadership   70
    1.2 Social responsibility   50
2. *Strategic Planning*
    2.1 Strategy development   40
    2.2 Strategy deployment   45
3. *Focus on Patients, Other Customers, and Markets*
    3.1 Patient, other customer, and healthcare market knowledge   40
    3.2 Patient and other customer relationships and satisfaction   45
4. *Measurement, Analysis, and Knowledge Management*
    4.1 Measurement and analysis of organizational performance   45
    4.2 Information and knowledge of management   45
5. *Staff Focus*
    5.1 Work systems   35
    5.2 Staff learning and motivation   25
    5.3 Staff well-being and satisfaction   25
6. *Process Management*
    6.1 Healthcare process   50
    6.2 Support processes   35
7. *Organizational Performance Results*
    7.1 Healthcare results   75
    7.2 Patient and other customer-focused results   75
    7.3 Financial and market results   75
    7.4 Staff and work system results   75
    7.5 Organizational effectiveness results   75
    7.6 Governance and social responsibility results   75

Source: Baldrige National Quality Program. 2004b. "Score Summary Worksheet,
Health Care Criteria." [Online information; retrieved 6/1/04.] www. quality.nist.gov/
PDF_files/2004_Scorebook_Full_Version.pdf.

The case study in the next section illustrates how using the Baldrige
criteria can jumpstart an organization's improvement process, provide
an impetus for favorable culture change, and elevate the financial and
clinical outcomes of the enterprise.

BEST PRACTICE CASE STUDY: SSM HEALTH CARE

Between 1988 and 2002, only 49 organizations received the Baldrige Award. In 2002, the first Baldrige Award was given to a healthcare provider—SSM Health Care[1] based in St. Louis, Missouri. At the same time, SSMHC was also selected as a Solucient 100 Top Hospital. This double distinction is a rare achievement and had never before been accomplished by any healthcare organization.

The story of SSMHC's 12-year corporate and hospital journey to achieve the Baldrige status is both thrilling and inspiring. In 1990, under the direction of its president and CEO Sr. Mary Jean Ryan, FSM, SSMHC began a systemwide implementation of continuous quality improvement (CQI), making SSMHC among the first Catholic-sponsored healthcare systems in the nation to do so. The organization's leaders found strong parallels between the values of SSMHC and the principles of CQI. SSMHC embraced CQI as a way to fulfill its mission. According to SSMHC's press releases, "While some health care organizations, desiring immediate results, abandoned CQI during the 1990s, SSM Health Care committed itself to a long-term journey. The system's leadership recognized that cultural change was required, which would take time."

In 1995, SSMHC began a systemwide process of applying for the Baldrige Award as a "fast track" to organizational excellence. SSMHC hospitals applied for state quality awards, while the system as a whole submitted its first Baldrige application in 1999. (For a complete look at SSMHC's Baldrige application, visit the system's web site at www.ssmhc.com.) SSMHC won several statewide quality awards between 1996 and 2001. In 1999, the system became the first healthcare organization in the country to receive a Baldrige site visit. Although it did not win right away, SSMHC applied three more times in the following years. The system pursued the award because its goal was to use the Baldrige criteria to improve the quality of services to patients. Using the Baldrige criteria raised SSMHC's standard of care at every one of its facilities.

SSMHC uses the Baldrige criteria to develop better approaches to patient care as well as to improve overall operations. For example, physicians at SSMHC hospitals work together using an innovative model called "Clinical Collaboratives" to focus on a specific healthcare area that demonstrates a need for improvement. The goal of the Clinical Collaboratives is to offer the best possible care to patients, one of the goals that differentiates SSMHC and that confirms its focus to embody a best-practice model.

In accepting the award, Sr. Mary Jean Ryan stated that "although the MBNQA is a significant milestone, the award is one component of SSMHC's 12-year continuous quality improvement efforts, which are ongoing across the system and in its individual entities." Still, she added, "the Baldrige model has been instrumental in helping us achieve our mission, because we have been using it for seven and a half years to improve the care we provide to those we serve."

The commitment made in 1990 by SSMHC focused on CQI and assessment of progress using the Baldrige criteria. This transformed the system's culture into one where *teamwork, continuous learning, innovation, breakthrough performance, and systems thinking* occur. This new culture is also characterized by a high level of consensus building and decision making, which yield the greatest impact and assign the greatest responsibility to all involved.

SSMHC's CQI journey led to significant improvements in all aspects of the health system throughout the 1990s. As acknowledged at that time by U.S. Department of Health and Human Services Secretary Tommy Thompson, "SSM Health Care's work with patient feedback and physician communications make it an outstanding example of what can be done when fresh thinking and modern science are brought to the delivery of health care in America. With its groundbreaking automated system that makes clinical information available to any of its physicians wherever they may be, SSM Health Care has shown that it is truly dedicated to bringing the technological revolution to health care. That's not just good for patients—it's good for our communities, and it's good for the health care industry at large."

Four of the major improvement outcomes achieved by SSMHC over its 12-year CQI journey and its 7-year Baldrige efforts are as follows:

1. In 1999, SSMHC formed four teams to start the Clinical Collaborative program. By 2002, this number had grown to 85 teams working on six clinical collaboratives.
2. The number of physicians connected to an automated information system has increased steadily, from 3,200 in 1999 to 7,288 in 2002.
3. For four consecutive years, SSMHC has maintained an investment AA credit rating—a rating attained by fewer than 1 percent of U.S. hospitals.

FIGURE 3.3 SSM HEALTH CARE'S PLANNING PROCESS

Initial Review
1. Vision statement
2. Mission statement
3. Data collection (continuous)
4. Data analysis (continuous)

Strategy Development
5. Environmental and market assessment
6. Internal assessment
7. Articulation of desired future
8. Setting goals and objectives
9. Identification of strategic options
10. Selection of specific strategies
11. Establishment of goals, objectives, and strategies for the next three years

Annual Operating Plans
12. Development of action plans
13. Analysis of impacts on volumes and financial performance
14. Development of capital project proposal
15. Capital allocation council meeting
16. Putting money and strategies together

Approval and Consolidation
17. Corporate staff review
18. Simultaneous development of detailed plans and budget among individual entities
19. System management review
20. Board approval
21. Approval of strategic and financial plans
22. Communication of plan
23. Implementation of plan
24. Monitoring of progress
25. Modification of plan as necessary

Source: Used with permission from SSM Health Care, St. Louis, Missouri.

4. In the past three years, SSMHC's share of the St. Louis market has increased by 18 percent; three of its competitors lost market share.

These are impressive outcomes, and most of them were achieved through the setting, monitoring, and reporting of metrics-driven goals.

Like all well-run and well-managed companies, SSMHC bases its operational decisions on a formal planning process, beginning with a three-year strategic plan. This plan is then quantified into a ten-year financial plan, which is ultimately used in each SSMHC hospital.

Figure 3.3 summarizes the many steps in SSMHC's planning process. As the figure shows, the organization's formal planning process involves 25 major steps. SSMHC has developed and uses this business-oriented methodology because it is aware that a formal process of determining its future state is dependent on research and analysis. In fact, SSMHC's strategic, financial, and human resources planning process (SFFP) combines, consolidates, and coordinates direction setting, strategy development, human resources, and financial planning. The SFFP ensures that SSMHC's networks and entities set strategic goals that are clearly oriented toward performance improvement. In fact, the process allows for the development of strategic objectives, system action plans, and key indicators in a systematic manner. Table 3.3 illustrates the synchronization of the objectives with the plans to develop specific indicators (metrics) for the entire system.

Other steps are involved in the planning process, but the focus here is on the metrics that SSMHC uses to produce Baldrige and 100 Top Hospitals results. These metrics are developed at both the system and individual hospital levels. Then, they are reported at various time periods to specific leadership forums for review. Decisions are made based on the metric outcomes relative to goals. Table 3.4 is a matrix of the reports that are periodically reviewed. The key elements of this matrix are the 16 systemwide performance review indicators (PIR) and the 49 hospital-developed PIRs.

Table 3.5 (page 68) shows the 16 systemwide PIRs along with the goals established for the 2002 budget year. SSMHC's individual entities report their actual values on a monthly basis through the 16 PIRs. If an unfavorable variance occurs beyond an established performance threshold in any of the system indicators, the entity is required to implement a corrective action plan using a standard format. Corrective analyses are used to prioritize opportunities for improvement or innovation at all levels of the organization. This way, SSMHC ensures that performance-monitoring results are turned into action plans for improvement if goals are not met.

TABLE 3.3 SSM HEALTH CARE'S STRATEGIC OBJECTIVES, SYSTEM ACTION PLANS, AND KEY INDICATORS

Strategic Objectives	System Action Plans (2002)	Key Indicators
Exceptional clinical outcomes	• Use Clinical Collaboratives to improve healthcare outcomes • Ensure patient safety	• Unplanned readmission rates • Medication event rate • Dangerous abbreviations
Exceptional patient, employee, and physician satisfaction	• Improve patient satisfaction with pain management • Implement Nursing Shared Accountability Model • Increase diversity representation with leadership	• Inpatient loyalty • Nurse turnover rate • Physician satisfaction • Employee satisfaction • Number of minorities in managerial, professional ranks
Exceptional financial performance	• Increase revenues and reduce expenses • Achieve growth • Reduce financial support to employed physicians • Improve staff productivity amid labor pressures • Improve medical management	• Operating margin percentage • Operating revenue per adjusted patient days • Expense per adjusted patient days • Admissions • Net revenue per physician • Paid hours/adjusted patient days • Average length of stay

Source: Used with permission from SSM Health Care, St. Louis, Missouri.

In addition to the systemwide PIR, each hospital is required to report, on a monthly basis, the results of 49 specific metrics that have been developed across the system to reveal the differences between the goals and the actual results (see Table 3.6 on page 69). This hospital-wide operational PIR is designed to monitor those metrics that are considered most important to the success of the individual hospitals. Most of the 16 PIRs are contained in the reports along with a number of metrics deemed critical to sustaining operational excellence. These 49 indicators are arrayed across influential success factor categories that include the following:

TABLE 3.4 SSM HEALTH CARE'S LEADERSHIP REVIEW FORUM: MONITORED REPORTS

Forum	Frequency	Reports Monitored	Purposes
SSMHC board of directors	• Quarterly • Annually • Annually	• Financial condition of the system • Healthy Communities report • Corporate Responsibilities Process (CRP) and Health Insurance Portability and Accountability Act (HIPAA) reports	2 2,3,4,5 5
Regional boards	• Quarterly	• Quarterly reports • Competency reports • CRP and HIPAA reports	3,4,5 3,4,5 5
System management	• Monthly • Monthly • Quarterly	• Network-entity combined financial statements • SSMHC performance indicator report (PIR) (16 indicators)/quality report • Quarterly ranking report (patient loyalty)	2 1,2,3,4 2,4
Operations council	• Monthly	• SSMHC PIR (16 indicators) • Network-entity combined financial statements • Entity variance report • Hospital PIR (49 indicators) • Corrective action plans: PIR/ quality report	1,2,3,4 2 2 1,2,3,4 2,5
Innsbrook Group	• Twice a year	• Network-entity combined financial statements	1,2,3,4
Network leadership/ entity administrative council	• Monthly • Quarterly	• Network-entity combined financial statements • Hospital PIR (49 indicators) • Entity quality report • Corrective action plans: PIR/quality report • Complaint report	2 1,2,3,4 3,4,5 2,5 3,4

Purposes: 1 = competitive performance; 2 = performance plan review; 3 = changing needs evaluation; 4 = organizational success; 5 = regulatory compliance
Source: Used with permission from SSM Health Care, St. Louis, Missouri.

TABLE 3.5 SSM HEALTH CARE'S 16 SYSTEM-LEVEL
PERFORMANCE INDICATOR REPORT, 2002

System-Level Indicators	Goal
• Inpatient loyalty index	54.5%
• Operating margin percentage	2.3%
• 31-day unplanned readmission rate	4.4%
• Acute admissions	37,614
• Employee satisfaction	N/A
• Physician satisfaction	N/A
• Prevalence of daily physical restraints	8%
• Home care patient loyalty index	64%
• Unrestricted days cash on hand	220
• Patient revenue per adjusted patient day (APD)	$1,331
• Operating expenses per APD	$1,315
• Operating margin percentage (hospitals)	4.5%
• Operating margin percentage (skilled nursing)	< 3%
• Operating margin percentage (home health)	9.6%
• Net revenue per physician	$31,407
• Practice direct operating cost percentage	70.9%

Source: Used with permission from SSM Health Care, St. Louis, Missouri.

- Growth
- Reimbursement
- Productivity/expense
- Liquidity
- Service and quality
- Employee satisfaction
- Profitability

Finally, hospital administrators at each SSMHC facility have developed daily operating reports that allow them to monitor the outcomes of several of the goals. These reports help to ensure that the biweekly, monthly, and quarterly goals that have been established at the corporate level will be achieved. Hospital leadership, particularly at the COO level and the operational vice presidents, peruse these daily reports for signs of variance from the goals, which, if necessary, will be corrected immediately. As this practice indicates, goals are more likely to be achieved when daily monitoring takes place. Figure 3.4 (page 72) is an

| | Current Month | | | | | | | Year to Date | | | | |
| | | | | Budget Variance | | Prior-Year Variance | | | | | Budget Variance | |
	Actual	Budget	Prior Year	Amount	Percent	Amount	Percent	Actual	Budget	Prior Year	Amount	Percent
Growth Indicators												
Acute admissions*	1,092	1,119	1,058	(27)	-2.4	34	3.2	6,735	6,923	6,784	(188)	-2.7
Acute patient days	4,850	4,925	4,572	(75)	-1.5	278	6.1	29,760	30,475	30,168	(715)	-2.3
Acute LOS	4.4	4.4	4.3	(0.0)	-0.9	(0.1)	-2.8	4.4	4.4	4.4	(0.0)	-0.4
Acute CMI	1.39	1.43	1.38	(0.03)	-2.3	0.02	1.1	1.43	1.41	1.41	0.02	1.1
Skilled admissions	0	0	0	0	0.0	0	0.0	0	0	0	0	0.0
Skilled patient days	0	0	0	0	0.0	0	0.0	0	0	0	0	0.0
Skilled LOS	N/A	N/A	N/A	N/A	N/A	N/A	N/A	N/A	N/A	N/A	N/A	N/A
Inpatient surgeries	389	427	381	(38)	-8.9	8	2.1	2,376	2,606	2,531	(230)	-8.8
Outpatient surgeries	537	513	495	24	4.7	42	8.5	3,009	2,928	2,872	81	2.8
Outpatient visits	4,379	5,451	4,999	(1,072)	-19.7	(620)	-12.4	28,179	32,563	31,953	(4,384)	-13.5
ER visits	2,972	3,199	2,182	(227)	-7.1	790	36.2	17,997	18,748	13,774	(751)	-4.0
Births	88	84	81	4	4.8	7	8.6	485	472	474	13	2.8
Reimbursement Indicators												
Reimbursement %	31.8%	32.5%	37.6%	-0.7%	-2.1	-5.8%	-15.4	31.7%	31.6%	35.4%	0.2%	0.5
Patient revenue per APD*	1,737	1,735	1,614	3	0.2	123	7.6	1,731	1,695	1,536	36	2.1
Bad debts and charity %	11.9%	11.3%	10.5%	-0.7%	-6.0	-1.4%	-13.6	12.9%	11.6%	10.7%	-1.3%	-11.0
Medicare admissions – traditional – med/surg	512	501	449	11	2.2	63	14.0	2,772	3,101	2,954	(329)	-10.6
Medicare CMI – traditional – med/surg	1.65	1.71	1.63	(0.06)	-3.3	0.02	1.4	1.71	1.67	1.67	0.04	2.1
Medicare LOS – traditional – med/surg	5.5	5.4	5.3	(0.0)	-0.8	(0.2)	-4.3	5.8	5.4	5.5	(0.3)	-5.7
Medicare admissions – managed – med/surg	0	54	53	(54)	-100.0	(53)	-100.0	160	332	449	(172)	-51.8
Medicare CMI – managed – med/surg	N/A	1.53	1.98	N/A	N/A	N/A	N/A	1.53	1.53	1.52	0.00	0.2
Medicare LOS – managed – med/surg	N/A	4.2	5.5	N/A	N/A	N/A	N/A	5.5	4.2	4.0	(1.3)	-31.8
Medicare traditional % gross patient revenue	51.3%	46.9%	44.9%	4.4%	9.5	6.4%	14.3	47.7%	47.3%	45.3%	0.4%	0.9
Medicare managed % gross patient revenue	0.1%	5.0%	6.3%	-5.0%	-98.2	-6.2%	-98.6	2.8%	5.0%	5.7%	-2.3%	-44.9
Medicaid % gross patient revenue	12.7%	10.3%	11.5%	2.4%	23.4	1.3%	11.1	12.5%	10.3%	11.2%	2.2%	21.1
Commercial managed % gross patient revenue	29.8%	31.0%	29.9%	-1.2%	-3.8	-0.2%	-0.6	31.3%	30.7%	30.9%	0.6%	1.9
Other % gross patient revenue	6.1%	6.8%	7.4%	-0.7%	-10.4	-1.3%	-17.7	5.7%	6.7%	6.9%	-1.0%	-14.2

(continued on following page)

TABLE 3.6 (continued)

Productivity/Expense Indicators												
Hospital FTEs (includes allocated)	1,154.9	1,174.0	1,161.3	19.1	1.6	6.4	0.6	1,157.3	1,160.4	1,225.4	3.2	0.3
Contract FTEs	43.2	40.8	53.8	(2.4)	-5.9	10.6	19.7	43.9	35.4	62.0	(8.5)	-24.1
Total FTEs (hospital+contract)	1,198.0	1,214.8	1,215.1	16.7	1.4	17.0	1.4	1,201.2	1,195.8	1,287.4	(5.4)	-0.4
Total paid hours/APD	30.4	29.6	31.8	(0.8)	-2.8	1.3	4.2	29.9	29.1	31.4	(0.8)	-2.7
Average hourly rate	29.3	29.9	28.7	0.6	2.1	(0.6)	-2.1	29.7	29.4	27.9	(0.2)	-0.8
Overtime %	1.6%	1.7%	1.8%	0.1%	4.1	0.1%	6.3	1.8%	1.8%	2.2%	0.0%	1.1
Compensation per APD	892	886	912	(7)	-0.8	20	2.2	888	857	879	(31)	-3.6
Supply expense per APD	387	324	358	(62)	-19.2	(28)	-7.9	361	330	350	(31)	-9.5
Operating expense per APD	1,810	1,724	1,798	(85)	-5.0	(12)	-0.7	1,828	1,712	1,705	(116)	-6.8
Liquidity Indicators												
Net days in accounts receivable	69.6	60.1	71.9	(9.6)	-15.9	2.2	3.1	69.6	60.1	71.9	(9.6)	-15.9
Unrestricted days cash on hand	(0.9)	14.9	18.7	(15.8)	-105.7	(19.6)	-104.5	(0.8)	15.0	18.5	(15.8)	-105.5
Service and Quality Indicators												
Inpatient loyalty index**	81.1%	82.3%	82.9%	-1.3%	-1.5	-1.8%	-2.2	81.7%	82.3%	81.9%	0.6%	-0.8
ER patient loyalty index	82.6%	77.2%	87.4%	5.4%	7.0	-4.8%	-5.5	77.7%	77.2%	76.4%	0.5%	0.6
Outpatient surgery loyalty index	87.6%	91.0%	89.9%	-3.4%	-3.7	-2.3%	-2.6	89.4%	91.0%	90.0%	-1.6%	-1.8
31-day acute readmission rate**	15.81%	11.50%	5.74%	-4.31%	-37.5	-10.07%	-175.4	10.46%	11.50%	4.91%	1.04%	9.0
Unscheduled returns to ER	1.79%	2.02%	2.06%	0.23%	11.4	0.27%	13.1	1.74%	2.02%	2.13%	0.28%	13.9
Unscheduled returns to OR	0.18%	0.67%	1.08%	0.49%	73.1	0.90%	83.3	0.29%	0.67%	0.77%	0.38%	56.7
Employee Satisfaction Indicators												
Employee satisfaction indicator**	N/A	73.00%	N/A	N/A	N/A	N/A	N/A	N/A	73.00%	N/A	N/A	N/A
Physician satisfaction indicator**	N/A	82.00%	N/A	N/A	N/A	N/A	N/A	N/A	82.00%	N/A	N/A	N/A
Profitability Indicators												
Operating revenue per AEA	5,687	5,461	5,262	226	4.1	426	8.1	5,517	5,415	5,037	102	1.9
Operating expense per AEA	5,764	5,319	5,636	(445)	-8.4	(129)	-2.3	5,665	5,346	5,381	(319)	-6.0
Operating margin %*	-1.4%	2.6%	-7.1%	-4.0%	-151.5	5.8%	81.0	-2.7%	1.3%	-6.8%	-4.0%	-310.2
Operating EBITDA %	3.9%	7.8%	-0.3%	-3.9%	-50.1	4.2%	1315.6	2.7%	6.8%	0.1%	-4.1%	-60.4

LOS: length of stay; APD: adjusted patient days; CMI: case mix index; FTE: full-time equivalent; AEA: adjusted equivalent admissions;

EBITDA: earnings before interest, taxes, depreciation, and amortization

* Systemwide indicator—requires corrective action plan if unfavorable variance to year-to-date plan exceeds 5%

** Systemwide indicator—measured in March and September, requires corrective action if year-to-date variance exceeds 70% loyalty, 60% clinical, and 60% satisfaction

Source: Used with permission from SSM Health Care, St. Louis, Missouri.

example of a daily operating report received by SSMHC's hospital leadership. Administrators at various hospitals rely greatly on the information generated in these daily reports. Without them, monthly goals are unlikely to be achieved.

The key to SSMHC's success is its strength in (1) developing metric goals that fully support its strategic plan and (2) monitoring and reporting the outcome of these goals across all of its hospitals to ensure that they are met or, if not met, at least positioned to be met in the near future. Essentially, SSMHC has taken a business approach within its not-for-profit tax-exempt grouping, deciding that it is best to achieve a set of goals that will push it beyond average outcomes and into, arguably, a position that will appeal to its broad constituency and customer base.

This success is all based on metric indicators that can be compared and benchmarked.

Benchmarking Methods That Work

SSMHC uses comparative information, both competitive and benchmark, to improve overall performance. Comparative information enables the system to assess its performance relative to that of similar organizations and to set stretch goals.

The need and priority for comparative data can be determined by answering *yes* to these questions:

- Does the comparative/benchmarking effort relate to the strategies and action plans of the strategic planning and financial planning processes?
- Are the data available and reliable?
- Does the comparative/benchmarking effort relate to the department-level indicators?

For SSMHC, sources of appropriate comparative information and data or benchmarking partners include the following:

- Organizations similar in size or providing similar services (e.g., healthcare systems)
- Organizations that compete in SSMHC markets
- Organizations known to excel at their comparison/benchmarking process

FIGURE 3.4 SSM HEALTH CARE'S DAILY HOSPITAL OPERATING SUMMARY

August	Births*	Pediatric Admissions + SCN (sick babies)	Adult Admissions	Adult + Pediatric + SCN Admissions	Midnight Census	Cumulative Length of Stay	Emergency Department Visits (based on charges posted)*	Outpatient Registrations*	Inpatient Surgeries*	Outpatient Surgeries*	Total Surgeries	Open-Heart Surgeries	Cardiac Catheterizations	Inpatient Revenue	Outpatient Revenue
1	1	0	43	43	163	3.79	104	199	24	18	42	1	20	1,172,443	506,876
Saturday 2	3	2	42	44	149	3.59	80	40	6	1	7	0	1	602,849	129,647
Sunday 3	4	1	14	15	134	4.37	74	24	5	0	5	0	0	435,716	139,252
4	4	1	54	55	168	3.91	105	229	20	28	48	3	14	1,109,287	657,494
5	0	2	42	44	175	3.93	89	188	16	15	31	2	7	1,116,312	433,525
6	1	2	42	44	161	3.88	114	184	13	17	30	1	12	828,066	440,992
7	3	1	35	36	154	3.93	81	203	8	35	43	3	8	817,852	488,775
8	0	3	42	45	156	3.87	112	176	19	18	37	4	14	1,130,889	514,028
Saturday 9	3	1	20	21	124	3.99	95	51	5	1	6	0	0	451,820	104,396
Sunday 10	1	0	13	13	122	4.18	106	18	4	0	4	0	0	413,090	205,454
11	1	0	52	52	157	4.04	102	201	16	21	37	1	7	1,073,455	389,687
Month-to-date actuals	21	13	399	412	1,663	4.04	1,062	1,513	136	154	290	15	83	9,151,778	4,010,125
Month-to-date budget	31			430	1,893	4.40	1,222	2,045	164	186	351			10,111,295	4,117,665
Variance	-10			-18	-230	0.37	-160	-532	-28	-32	-61			-959,517	-107,539
% variance	-31.2%			-4.2%	-12.2%	8.3%	-13.1%	-26.0%	-17.2%	-17.3%	-17.3%			-9.5%	-2.6%
Month budget	86			1,212	5,335	4.4018152	3,444	5,762	463	525				28,495,468	11,604,328

Source: Used with permission from SSM Health Care, St. Louis, Missouri.

In addition, SSMHC uses the International Benchmarking Clearinghouse's four-step benchmarking process (SSMHC 2004):

Step 1: *Plan the study*. Form a sharing network, decide what to benchmark, and determine how information will be collected and shared.

Step 2: *Collect information*. Collect information about a successful comparison process, seek out benchmarking partners, and investigate how superior performance is achieved by other organizations.

Step 3: *Analyze results*. Compare the organization's own practices to that of other organizations, examine the findings for gaps between practices, and uncover innovative approaches to close gaps.

Step 4: *Adapt and improve*. Adapt the best practice or implement specific improvements to existing process and measure results after implementation.

In conclusion, each hospital or health system has an opportunity to extend SSMHC's business approach to its facilities. It does not take a lot more effort to begin this process, but it does take dedicated leadership and a strong commitment to improvement. So many opportunities are available for moving toward best practices.

Although he was not aware of it, Sam Barnes was in luck. Pleasant Flats Medical Center was undergoing a CQI effort and had adopted portions of a metrics-based management system that focuses on various goals, including clinical outcomes. Unbeknown to Sam, one of these clinical goals was, "unplanned returns to the emergency department." For this goal, management had implemented a number of processes and procedures to ensure that patients were properly treated the first time through. As a result, the time it took for a patient to be seen and treated (patient throughput) was decreased and patient outcomes had improved through use of better diagnostic tools and capable, trained employees.

These measures resulted in Sam's successful visit to Pleasant Flats's ER. Sam was evaluated, triaged, treated, and released in a timely manner. He returned to his life and came away from his ER experience with very favorable opinions of the hospital, an opinion he planned to share with everyone he met.

REFERENCES

Baldrige National Quality Program. 2004a. "Getting Started with the Criteria for Performance Excellence: A Guide to Self-Assessment and Action." [Online information; retrieved 6/1/04.] http://www.quality.nist.gov/Getting_Started.htm.

———. 2004b. "Score Summary Worksheet, Health Care Criteria." [Online information; retrieved 6/1/04.] http://www.quality.nist.gov/PDF_files/2004_Scorebook_Full_Version.pdf.

Griffith, J., and J. Alexander. 2002. "Measuring Comparative Hospital Performance." *Journal of Healthcare Management* 47 (1): 41–57.

Harrington, H. J., and J. S. Harrington. 1996. *High Performance Benchmarking: 20 Steps to Success.* New York: McGraw Hill.

SSM Health Care. 2004. "Comparative Data." [Online information; retrieved 6/1/04.] http://www.ssmhc.com/internet/home/ssmcorp.nsf/Documents/ED1FE6BA322D0E9A86256C7600528A13?OpenDocument.

Walton, S. (with John Huey). 1992. *Made in America*, 63. New York: Doubleday.

NOTE

1. Information on SSM Health Care was obtained with permission.

PRACTICAL TIPS

☛ Adopt benchmarking as a management technique. Investigate the various proprietary hospital-benchmarking services, and select the one that meets the needs of your organization. Make sure to choose a service that employs a reputable and verifiable method of goal setting and comparison.

☛ Recognize the current metric indicators being used by the 100 Top Hospitals (see www.solucient.com), and develop action plans relating to these indicators to improve your organization's outcomes—financially, operationally, and clinically.

☛ Review the Malcolm Baldrige Criteria for Performance Excellence, and determine if your hospital is in position or can be put in position to begin the journey toward clinical and financial improvement.

CHAPTER FOUR

Establishing the Use of Balanced Scorecards to Improve Goal Setting and Monitoring

Pleasant Flats Medical Center had a challenge. Earlier in the year, its CEO, Jon Taylor, learned more about peer-group benchmarking at a seminar and became convinced of the reliability of using median and percentile ranks in setting goals for the organization. Jon knew that several improvement opportunities were available to Pleasant Flats, so he directed the leadership group to seek them out and set goals to capture them. Although the leadership group worked diligently toward this assignment, the leaders were relatively stumped on how to present the information they found in a manner that would signal that the goals were being met. Jon asked the hospital CFO, Jane Zabrowsky, to develop a methodology that would allow Pleasant Flats to understand its outcomes in a concise way.

"Jon," said Jane, "I will work on it and see what I can do. I have been hearing about a process that might help us do what you want. Let me check it out and get back to you."

"Okay, Jane, but let's make it snappy," Jon replied. "Now that I see the kinds of improvements possible with good information, I want to see them happen as soon as possible."

IN CHAPTER 2, in our discussion of methods for presenting information in a meaningful way, the balanced scorecard is put forth as a useful technique to significantly improve organizational outcomes.

FIGURE 4.1 BALANCED SCORECARD OUTCOMES

- Strategy that is clear and has gained consensus
- Strategy that is communicated throughout the organization
- Departmental and personal goals that are aligned with the strategy
- Strategic objectives that are linked to long-term targets and annual budgets
- Strategic initiatives that are identified and aligned
- Strategic reviews that are performed periodically and systematically
- Feedback that can be used to learn about and improve strategy

In this chapter, we further examine the balanced scorecard concept, which can be used to set goals and to monitor and report results.

WHAT IS THE BALANCED SCORECARD?

According to Robert Kaplan and David Norton (1996), authors of the classic business text *The Balanced Scorecard*, the scorecard is a means to translate an organization's mission and strategy into a comprehensive set of performance measures, providing the framework for a strategic measurement and management system. The balanced scorecard measures organizational performance across four balanced perspectives:

1. Financial
2. Customers
3. Internal business processes
4. Learning and growth

The use of these four aggregate measures enables an organization to track financial results while simultaneously monitoring progress in building the capabilities and acquiring the intangible assets needed for future growth. Further, the organization can retain an emphasis on achieving financial objectives by including the metrics that drive the performance of these financial objectives in its outcomes. Figure 4.1 summarizes the benefits that can be expected when the balanced scorecard is adopted.

The balanced scorecard is a relatively new (started in the 1990s) management tool. It has been receiving positive press for its ability to help an organization establish strategic direction (goals) and develop specific action plans to achieve these goals. Further, after the organization implements its action plans, the balanced scorecard tool assists in creating a superior methodology for monitoring the results of the activities.

Pioneered in the manufacturing sector to generate value-added information for business leaders, the balanced scorecard is increasingly relied on by healthcare organizations to perform the same function for them. Beyond allowing leaders to align their strategies to their organization's mission and vision statements, the balanced scorecard also communicates a more specific set of requirements to enterprise stakeholders. As Kaplan and Norton (1996, 21) states, "The Balanced Scorecard retains financial measurement as a critical summary of managerial and business performance, but it highlights a more general and integrated set of measurements that link customer, internal process, employee, and system performance to long-term financial success."

Measurement of performance in the four areas of focus—financial, customers, internal business processes, and learning and growth—results in a natural and continuous feedback loop, which then offers continual improvement possibilities to an organization. An organization may use different performance measures within these four quadrants. Figure 4.2 highlights several objectives for each quadrant that can and should be developed by an organization for its own scorecard. As Kaplan and Norton reveal in their research, almost any organization that moves to maximize the results within the three nonfinancial areas (e.g., setting high goals for customer satisfaction, internal operations, and learning and growth) will find a natural and often quite substantial improvement in its financial quadrant.

How to Develop a Balanced Scorecard

A balanced scorecard can be developed in a number of ways. However, a good methodology would include the following actions:

1. *Develop an executable business strategy.* Determine the important objectives of the organization, and base the strategy on those goals. This process entails finding out what key performance

FIGURE 4.2 BALANCED SCORECARD QUADRANT OBJECTIVES

Financial
- Return on capital
- Competitive position
- Growth in volume
- Reduced cash outlays
- Improved cash receipts

Customers
- Increased patient satisfaction
- Increased employee satisfaction
- Increased physician satisfaction

Internal Processes
- Product innovation
- Perfect orders (or error reduction)
- Improved clinical outcome
- Higher-quality indicators

Learning and Growth
- Strategic awareness
- Mandated hours of education per employee

---

indicators—whether financial, clinical, or satisfaction related—contribute the most to the success of the organization.

2. *Describe the strategy.* Assist those who are affected by and are responsible for implementing the organizational strategy in understanding the reasons behind it. This understanding leads to much greater buy-in. For example, hold meetings with key stakeholders, such as department managers, in which explanations are given as to why certain indicators were chosen and how these indicators make an impact on organizational outcomes.

3. *Design and develop the scorecard framework with performance metrics.* These metrics should closely follow the strategic objectives outlined by the organization.

This way, the scorecard is not just a set of unrelated metrics. It is a representation of the organization's system for setting financial and nonfinancial goals and for monitoring those goals to achieve preferred outcomes.

How to Balance the Scorecard

Not all metrics are equal. Some are more valuable to the organization's ultimate results than others. Thus, it is important to value these metrics and develop a weighting mechanism for the major categories. This way, the scorecard is "balanced" according to the metric's values.

The four quadrants of a balanced scorecard generally have a relative consistency, with no one quadrant being allocated a disproportionate share of the total resources of an organization. In contrast, an unbalanced scorecard allocates 70 percent of the total to the financial quadrant, leaving only 30 percent for the other three quadrants. While this type of allocation may have a short-term benefit, it could have a deleterious impact on the organization's financial and nonfinancial outcomes in the long run. A balanced approach, according to Kaplan and Norton (1996), allocates approximately 30 percent each to financial and internal processes and 20 percent each to customers and learning and growth.

BALANCED SCORECARDS IN HEALTHCARE

The healthcare industry, as any other industry, can benefit from using the balanced scorecard. Figure 4.3 illustrates the quadrants and aggregate objectives that can, and should, be used to measure performance for a hospital. As can be seen in the figure, the list of goals goes well beyond the financial indicators, allowing recipients of the report to gain a more complete insight into the goals and achievements of the organization.

The figure shows all of the highly critical indicators, signaling that it is crucial to set goals for each area, not just the financial category. In fact, excelling in the nonfinancial elements is likely to bring greater financial success than downplaying the nonfinancial elements. Figure 4.3 also shows the outcome score for each objective.

Scoring Grid

Healthcare Insights, LLC (see www.hcillc.com), a training and software development firm that specializes in tools and techniques for improving general and financial management for healthcare organizations,

FIGURE 4.3 EXAMPLE OF A HOSPITAL'S BALANCED SCORECARD

Perspectives

Financial (Aggregate Score)   2.01 Needs improvement

    Return on net assets   2.61 Good
    Competitive position   0.83 Unsatisfactory
    Growth in volume   1.50 Poor
    Reduced cash outlays   3.50 Good
    Improved cash receipts   1.62 Poor

Customers (Aggregate Score)   2.47 Needs improvement

    Patient satisfaction survey   2.20 Needs improvement
    Employee satisfaction survey   2.40 Needs improvement
    Physician satisfaction survey   2.80 Needs improvement

Internal Processes (Aggregate Score)   3.34 Good

    Product innovation   3.00 Good
    Error reduction   2.50 Needs improvement
    Quality indicators   4.10 Very good
    Clinical outcome   3.75 Good

Learning and Growth (Aggregate Score)   3.00 Good

    Strategic awareness   3.00 Good
    Leadership survey   3.20 Good
    Mandated hours of education per employee   2.80 Needs improvement

Overall Performance	Score	Weight	Weighted Score
Financial	2.01	0.35	0.704
Customers	2.47	0.20	0.493
Internal processes	3.34	0.30	1.001
Learning and growth	3.00	0.15	0.450
Total Score			2.649 Needs improvement

has developed an automated technique for valuing an organization's goals. This method scores the results in numbers, words, and colors.

The simple methodology compares an organization's actual results against benchmark percentile values. The scoring system, developed by Mary Grace Wilkus, chief software architect at Healthcare Insights,

TABLE 4.1 BALANCED SCORECARD SCORING METHODOLOGY

Description	Benchmark Percentile Rank	Score
Excellent	Top 10th	5
Very good	75th–89th	4
Good	50th–74th	3
Needs improvement	25th–49th	2
Poor	10th–24th	1
Unsatisfactory	Bottom 10th	0

Source: Used with permission from Healthcare Insights, LLC., 2004, Libertyville, Illinois.

allows the organization to use benchmarks in setting goals and monitoring results for the scorecard. Individual indicators are analyzed against the organization's own goals and against peer organizations to reveal how the organization is performing. These values can be obtained in several ways, including through rating agencies, proprietary benchmarking services, and other established peer standards. Table 4.1 delineates how Healthcare Insights's scoring system works.

This scoring methodology can yield a one-page result that states the organization's performance relative to the benchmark percentile ranks. No organization should be operating at less than the 50th percentile (also known as the median). Thus, according to the ranking methodology, any result less than 3 should be unacceptable, and corrective action plans should immediately be set in place. Further, the automated methodology provides an online component, whereby recipients of the results can instantly "drill down" or select (by clicking on) the applicable line for additional information. This additional information generally represents actual indicators that can be used to find the organization's ranks within the percentiles. Recipients can also learn the value of the indicators that are acceptable or unacceptable.

Table 4.2 represents an example of a drill down from the first-line item—return on net assets. In this case, the executive team at the hospital has determined that the indicators in the figure are most important to the organization's success and has incorporated these indicators into the hospital operations. The three major rating agencies—Standard &

TABLE 4.2 Balanced Scorecard Drill Down: Financial Perspective Aggregate Indicator, Return on Net Assets

Indicator	Positive Trend	Prior Year		Current Year		Compared to Benchmark	
		Month	Year to Date	Month	Year to Date	Score	Descriptor
Profitability						3.60	Good
Operating margin	Up	0.04	0.05	0.04	0.05	4.00	Very Good
Excess (total) margin	Up	0.07	0.08	0.11	0.13	5.00	Excellent
Earnings before interest, depreciation, and amortization (EBIDA)							
revenue	Up	0.18	0.16	0.17	0.16	3.00	Good
EBIDA assets	Up	0.08	0.07	0.12	0.11	3.00	Good
Return on equity	Up	0.09	0.07	0.09	0.08	3.00	Good
Liquidity						1.75	Poor
Days cash on hand (all sources)	Up	224.00	227.00	234.00	240.00	5.00	Excellent
Current	Up	1.1	1.1	1.2	1.2	1.00	Poor
Days of revenue in accounts receivable	Down	82.00	91.00	85.00	86.00	1.00	Poor
Average payment period	Down	110.00	112.00	105.00	107.00	0.00	Unsatisfactory
Capital Structure						1.60	Poor
Equity financing	Up	0.15	0.14	0.15	0.14	1.00	Poor
Long-term debt to capitalization	Down	0.72	0.72	0.71	0.72	2.00	Needs improvement
Cash flow to total debt	Up	0.04	0.03	0.04	0.03	1.00	Poor
Annual debt service coverage	Up	2.04	2.10	2.10	2.00	1.00	Poor
Cushion	Up	9.40	9.20	9.50	9.60	3.00	Good
Asset Efficiency						3.50	Good
Total asset turnover	Up	1.28	1.18	1.26	1.25	4.00	Very Good
Inventory turnover	Up	14	15	15	16	3.00	Good
Total Return on Net Assets						2.61	Needs improvement

Poor's, Moody's, and Fitch—use many financial indicators to do a financial analysis of hospitals. In this example, the hospital wants to monitor the same financial indicators used by external rating agencies.

Another drill-down example is represented in Table 4.3—improved cash receipts. In this example, 21 key revenue cycle metrics have been developed and aggregated by this author into the balanced scorecard drill down. The indicators used here are what the hospital believes to

TABLE 4.3 Balanced Scorecard Drill Down: Financial Perspective Aggregate Indicator, Improved Cash Receipts

	Prior Year		Current Year		Compared to Benchmark	
Indicator	Month	Year to Date	Month	Year to Date	Score	Descriptor
Number of total accounts on pre-bill edits	90	60	100	86	1.00	Poor
Dollars of total accounts on pre-bill edits	$45,000	$30,000	$50,000	$42,000	1.00	Poor
Number of total accounts on pre-bill edits as a % of total	9.0%	6.0%	10.0%	8.6%	1.00	Poor
Dollars of total accounts on pre-bill edits as a % of total	6.0%	4.0%	5.0%	5.5%	1.00	Poor
Number of denied claims	400	300	400	380	2.00	Needs improvement
Dollars of denied claims	$110,000	$60,000	$100,000	$105,000	2.00	Needs improvement
Patient satisfaction	85	90	83	86	2.00	Needs improvement
Registration error rates	25.0%	4.0%	20.0%	16.0%	1.00	Poor
Identified underpayments	6.0%	0.0%	4.2%	4.3%	2.00	Needs improvement
Collection of identified non-payments or underpayments	55.0%	100.0%	50.0%	60.0%	1.00	Poor
Gross days outstanding	78.0	65.0	75.0	75.0	1.00	Poor
Net days outstanding	78.0	65.0	80.0	80.0	1.00	Poor
Percentage of clean claims submitted	95.2%	95.0%	97.9%	98.0%	3.00	Good
Daily cash collections	$93,000	$95,000	$92,000	$94,500	2.00	Needs improvement
Collections as a % of net revenues	97.4%	100.0%	98.0%	98.7%	2.00	Needs improvement
Bad debt write-offs as a % of gross revenues	3.3%	3.0%	2.4%	2.3%	3.00	Good
Bad debt recoveries as a % of gross revenues	27.0%	25.0%	14.0%	20.0%	3.00	Good
Charity care write-off as a % of gross revenue	1.2%	2.0%	1.1%	0.9%	1.00	Poor
Gross credit balance days outstanding	3.1	2.0	3.3	3.0	1.00	Poor
Percentage of claims denied	5.0%	3.0%	4.6%	4.0%	1.00	Poor
Cost-to-collect ratio	3.0%	2.8%	3.0%	2.9%	2.00	Needs improvement
Total improved cash receipts					1.62	Poor

have the greatest impact on the revenue cycle process. Some of the indicator outcomes are related to specific revenue cycle benchmarks, where available. In other cases, the hospital has developed and/or extrapolated medians and percentiles that represent ranges of success.

Like the return on net assets indicators, these 21 revenue cycle indicators roll up into a single number that represents the organization's overall outcome for this important element of the balanced scorecard. In this way, the recipient of the report can determine, at a glance, the outcomes of the operation. This is another value-added method to enforce management accountability.

Other Issues

Two more issues should be mentioned if an organization is considering adopting a balanced scorecard methodology for goal setting and monitoring. The more choices that a hospital is aware of and can use in its operations, the more likely it is to successfully choose and implement these management techniques.

First, another goal-setting system is beginning to gain awareness within the healthcare industry. Known as the "Five Pillars," this system was developed by Quint Studer (see www.thestudergroup.com), a former hospital administrator who has become a management consultant and trainer. Like the balanced scorecard, the Five Pillars represent overarching elements of a hospital's operation. Studer (2003, 51), in his book *Hardwiring Excellence*, define the components of the Five Pillars: service, quality, people, finance, and growth.

Many individual indicators are suggested within each pillar, but the overall idea is to align organizational goals with the pillars. As Studer says, "We are not measuring just to measure. We are measuring to align specific leadership and employee behaviors that cascade throughout the organization to drive results" (2003, 61). That is exactly the right reason to develop the information-driven hospital. Measurement presents an opportunity to manage the modern medical center using metrics that show how outcomes can be improved.

Second, an organization that adopts a balanced scorecard approach should do so not only at the organizational level. If the hospital is really serious about using balanced scorecard metrics to improve its outcomes, then it should also adopt specific metric indicators at the departmental level. Departmental metrics are unit specific, related to the work, services, and performance of the stakeholders within that department. These metrics should be aligned with and support the organizationwide indicators, and managers must be completely aware of them and must be held accountable for their achievement. Selection of departmental metrics will determine whether the organization will be able to meet the goals it believes are important to its continued operation and existence.

Being aware of how your own organization is performing relative to its peers is extremely important because business is likely to be lost if performance is not monitored. The balanced scorecard is an excellent tool, helping accelerate excellence in management and providing the best opportunity for the organization to achieve its stated goals.

BALANCED SCORECARD CASE STUDY 1: BRIDGEPORT HOSPITAL

Bridgeport Hospital (BH)[1] is a 425-bed community teaching hospital. It is a member of Yale New Haven Health System and is affiliated with the Yale School of Medicine. Located in Bridgeport, Connecticut, a community with two hospitals, BH has always been interested in improving both its financial and clinical outcomes.

In the late 1990s, BH was an administratively driven organization operating with a silo mentality. Like many of its competitors, BH was coming off a failed capitation strategy that had decreased its revenue streams. The leadership at BH determined that the clinical department chairs were not fully engaged in operations of their services and the community physicians were going around the chairs to do as they pleased. At the same time, the hospital's financial condition was worsening. In fact, during this period, consultants recommended that the hospital downsize its operation.

From a monitoring and reporting perspective, BH was a classic example of how an organization uses indicators. The hospital only used a few clinical indicators, but most of the indicators it reported were financial. The CEO knew what he did not want to do, but he needed a framework for leadership.

Out of a series of meetings in the late 1990s, BH's leadership finally realized that setting and monitoring objectively determined metrics-based goals was a viable solution to several of the issues they were facing. In 1999, BH adopted the balanced scorecard concept and incorporated it as part of the organization's long-range planning process, which was termed Scenarios for Destination 2005.

FIGURE 4.4 BRIDGEPORT HOSPITAL'S BALANCED SCORECARD

Fiscal Year 2000 Strategic Imperatives

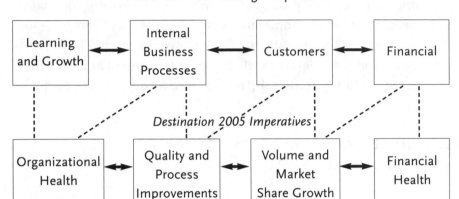

Source: Used with permission from Bridgeport Hospital, Bridgeport, Connecticut.

The balanced scorecard was constructed as a three-year phase-in project. In Year 1 (2000), BH used Kaplan and Norton's balanced scorecard four quadrants. However, the leadership later determined that the hospital metrics were "force fit" into the quadrants; the framework just "did not feel right," according to administrators. Because of this, the major elements of the Kaplan and Norton scorecard were changed in Year 2 (2001). Rather than remain uncomfortable with the fit of the four quadrants, BH created its own framework that accommodates five areas of indicators: organizational health, quality improvement, process improvement, market share growth, and financial health.

In Year 3 (2002), BH combined two of the five major areas of key indicators to return to a quadrants-based methodology. The four remaining major scorecard indicators were organizational health, quality and process improvements, volume and market share growth, and financial health. Figure 4.4 shows the development and change from the original set of aggregate measures in 2000 to the Destination 2005 imperatives.

One of the key lessons from the BH example is that although the balanced scorecard is an extremely useful tool, it can be amended according to an organization's needs. Modifying the main criteria is acceptable to achieve the results desired by an organization.

In developing its own methodologies for improvement, using the balanced scorecard model as a guide, BH determined that it needed to focus on three major operational areas: clinical inputs by the medical advisory board, performance management, and financial metrics.

Clinical Inputs by the Medical Advisory Board

As stated, BH faced significant physician issues. The department chairs were not fully engaged in the operation of their services, and many of the community physicians were not consulting with the department chairs to operate as they chose. Thus, hospital leadership determined that the key to driving change in this area was to develop a medical advisory board. The purpose of the panel was to solicit physician feedback and participation in establishing strategies for the hospital's future.

The formation of the medical advisory panel was riddled with not only territorial concerns but also anxiety over selection of the cochairs and participants and identification of the responsibility of the panel. In the end, the panel determined that a comprehensive educational process—involving training in finance, managed care, nursing, information technology management, and planning and marketing—was required of all panel members to ensure that everyone had the same basic knowledge. Staff support teams were assembled, spokespersons were identified and charged, and weekly meetings were held during the first six months to develop action and implementation plans.

The medical advisory board developed a number of themes and established goals around those themes. Each of the themes had numerical targets designed to move the hospital forward in the community. Figure 4.5 lists these major themes, which are very much oriented around the balanced scorecard approach.

The medical advisory panel met consistently over an 18-month period and achieved significant results. Some overarching outcomes include the following:

- Initiation of new clinical programs
- Adoption and implementation of protocols for the intensive care unit and drug administration
- Implementation of physician-to-physician marketing ideas
- Significant recruitment and retention systems for registered nurses, with vacancy rates aimed at less than 3 percent

FIGURE 4.5 BRIDGEPORT HOSPITAL'S MEDICAL ADVISORY
BOARD THEMES

- Patient service
- Marketing
- Growth
- Cost efficiency
- Clinical quality and patient safety
- Patient flow
- Operating room efficiencies

Source: Used with permission from Bridgeport Hospital, Bridgeport, Connecticut.

- Creation of bed-flow coordinator position to facilitate patient movement

Further, the physicians as a group benefited from the use of a medical advisory panel. Among these morale-boosting advantages were cross-pollination of ideas from the medical staff to administration/management, physician pride in their work toward the effort as the improvement processes began to take effect, and physician realization that their involvement in strategy setting and buy-in of the strategy are essential for financial success.

Performance Management

Another initiative undertaken by BH leadership was the development of a more organized approach to set priorities for and to manage clinical services. BH formed clinical program teams (CPTs) to focus on eight areas: diagnostic services, emergency services, Heart Institute, medicine, pediatrics, psychiatry, surgery and anesthesia, and women and maternity.

The CPTs were given authority, responsibility, structure, and support to set their own balanced scorecard goals for their respective areas (see Figure 4.6) and to work toward achieving those goals. Once measurable goals were established, monitoring the implementation actions became easy.

FIGURE 4.6 BRIDGEPORT HOSPITAL'S CLINICAL PROGRAM TEAMS

Authority

- Implements actions and plans as appropriate to meet targets within organization
- Decides to change course to achieve targets if change is budget neutral
- Works across the organization (breaks down silos)

Structure

- Is led by department chairs and senior staff; includes program area experts (e.g., physicians, nurses in rehabilitation, home care), information system, finance, quality, and planning and marketing
- Meets regularly
- Develops and implements actions in concert with overall plan, and achieves strategic performance measures

Responsibility

- Is fully responsible and accountable for achieving goals in
  - quality and process improvements,
  - volume growth,
  - market share,
  - cost reduction, and
  - revenue generation
- Stays current in clinical area
- Actively engages all levels of staff
- Shares ideas broadly
- Provides timely analysis and decision making
- Monitors progress concurrently, and reports on indicators monthly

Support

- Has access to data and information—key information databases on quality, volume, market share, profit/loss, and cost
- Is provided education on quality, financial, information systems, and planning and marketing along with staff support from these areas

Source: Used with permission from Bridgeport Hospital, Bridgeport, Connecticut.

Figure 4.7 shows examples of indicators developed by CPTs. From a balanced scorecard perspective, this figure clearly illustrates that the hospital was adhering to a comprehensive set of criteria to achieve its goals.

Outcomes

The CPTs were highly successful; they assisted the hospital in setting and achieving higher goals. Here are some of the outcomes they achieved:

- Clearer alignment of individual goals and overall organizational goals
- Balanced set of performance indicators
- Engagement of clinical leadership in organizational goals
- Breakdown of organizational silos
- Organizationwide adoption of an outcome focus, changing a culture of process to a culture of results

FIGURE 4.7 BRIDGEPORT HOSPITAL'S CLINICAL PROGRAM
TEAMS' INDICATORS

Organizational Health
- Attitude, skills, competencies, learning
- Employee and physician satisfaction rankings
- Turnover rates, vacancy rates

Quality and Process Improvements
- Cycle times, turnaround times, productivity
- "Door-to-floor" measures
- Lengths of stay
- Patient satisfaction levels
- Clinical outcomes (e.g., mortality, readmission, nosocomial infection)
- Customer perception

Volume and Market Share Growth
- Emergency department, outpatient and inpatient

Financial Health
- Operating margin
- Cost/case mix index adjusted equivalent discharge
- Net revenue/case mix index adjusted equivalent discharge
- Variable costs/case

Source: Used with permission from Bridgeport Hospital, Bridgeport, Connecticut.

Past Successes and Future Opportunities

Figure 4.8 lists BH's balanced scorecard indicators for 2002 and for the Destination 2005 imperative. This is an impressive and comprehensive set of indicators, highlighting the breadth and depth of the balanced scorecard and placing the indicators in a context of achievement.

As an outgrowth to its success in using the scorecard, BH evolved to the next level: in fiscal year 2004, BH's overall health system decided to adapt its scorecard concept. The leadership team set four key dimensions for the entire system to plan around: (1) employer of choice; (2) patient safety, quality, and operations improvement; (3) provider of choice; and (4) financial performance. The team then brainstormed overall system goals and measures within each of the key dimensions. Afterward, each local facility adopted the system goals and measures

	2002	2005
Organizational Health		
Turnover rate as a % of the national average	93.5%	80.0%
Vacancy rate as a % of the national average	93.5%	80.0%
Physician satisfaction percentile	Identify	90.0
Med/surg 1:6 nursing ratio maintained	90.0%	100.0%
Quality and Process Improvements		
Patient satisfaction percentile—inpatient	> 50.0	> 90.0
Patient satisfaction percentile—		
emergency department	> 23.0	> 90.0
Nosocomial pressure ulcers	< 3.3%	< 0.5%
Emergency department treat and		
release patient < 120 minutes	55.0%	70.0%
Emergency department patients		
admitted < 4 hours	40.0%	70.0%
Percentage of physician orders entered		
electronically	40.0%	90.0%
Volume and Market Share Growth		
Volume	20,329	20,738
Market share	> 24.4%	> 25.0%
Financial Health		
Operating margin	> 0.5%	> 3.0%

Source: Used with permission from Bridgeport Hospital, Bridgeport, Connecticut.

and added its own goals and measures. Figure 4.9 presents this concept visually.

Finally, BH realized the need to track key indicators in each dimension in real time so that the system can identify and respond to business changes proactively. As a result, BH formed a systemwide committee, which worked for more than a year to develop performance indicators and standard definitions and, with help from an outside software developer, to create an electronic balanced scorecard that is updated in real time and is accessible (via desk computers) to all key managers across the system.

FIGURE 4.9 BRIDGEPORT HOSPITAL'S FISCAL YEAR 2004 BUSINESS PLAN

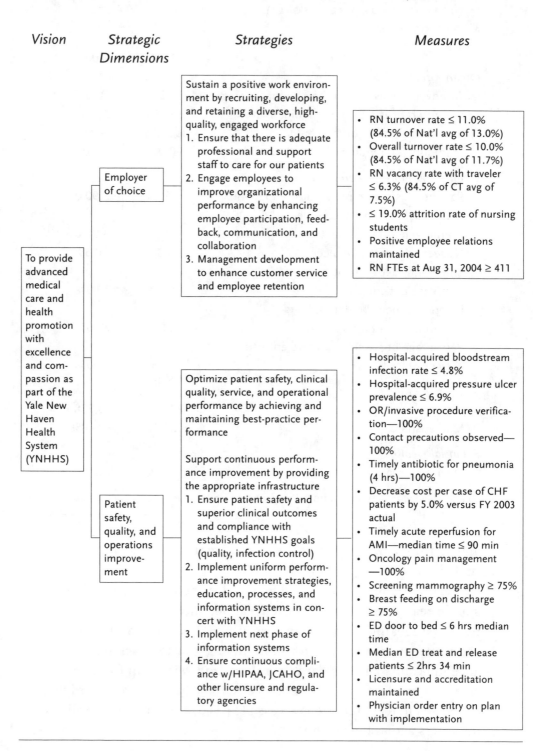

Vision	Strategic Dimensions	Strategies	Measures
To provide advanced medical care and health promotion with excellence and compassion as part of the Yale New Haven Health System (YNHHS)	Employer of choice	Sustain a positive work environment by recruiting, developing, and retaining a diverse, high-quality, engaged workforce 1. Ensure that there is adequate professional and support staff to care for our patients 2. Engage employees to improve organizational performance by enhancing employee participation, feedback, communication, and collaboration 3. Management development to enhance customer service and employee retention	• RN turnover rate ≤ 11.0% (84.5% of Nat'l avg of 13.0%) • Overall turnover rate ≤ 10.0% (84.5% of Nat'l avg of 11.7%) • RN vacancy rate with traveler ≤ 6.3% (84.5% of CT avg of 7.5%) • ≤ 19.0% attrition rate of nursing students • Positive employee relations maintained • RN FTEs at Aug 31, 2004 ≥ 411
	Patient safety, quality, and operations improvement	Optimize patient safety, clinical quality, service, and operational performance by achieving and maintaining best-practice performance Support continuous performance improvement by providing the appropriate infrastructure 1. Ensure patient safety and superior clinical outcomes and compliance with established YNHHS goals (quality, infection control) 2. Implement uniform performance improvement strategies, education, processes, and information systems in concert with YNHHS 3. Implement next phase of information systems 4. Ensure continuous compliance w/HIPAA, JCAHO, and other licensure and regulatory agencies	• Hospital-acquired bloodstream infection rate ≤ 4.8% • Hospital-acquired pressure ulcer prevalence ≤ 6.9% • OR/invasive procedure verification—100% • Contact precautions observed—100% • Timely antibiotic for pneumonia (4 hrs)—100% • Decrease cost per case of CHF patients by 5.0% versus FY 2003 actual • Timely acute reperfusion for AMI—median time ≤ 90 min • Oncology pain management—100% • Screening mammography ≥ 75% • Breast feeding on discharge ≥ 75% • ED door to bed ≤ 6 hrs median time • Median ED treat and release patients ≤ 2hrs 34 min • Licensure and accreditation maintained • Physician order entry on plan with implementation

FIGURE 4.9 *(continued)*

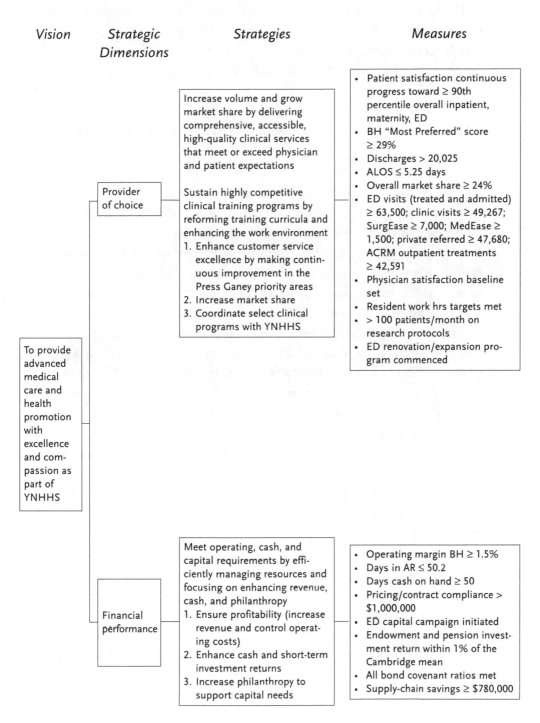

Vision	Strategic Dimensions	Strategies	Measures

Vision: To provide advanced medical care and health promotion with excellence and compassion as part of YNHHS

Strategic Dimensions — Provider of choice

Strategies:

Increase volume and grow market share by delivering comprehensive, accessible, high-quality clinical services that meet or exceed physician and patient expectations

Sustain highly competitive clinical training programs by reforming training curricula and enhancing the work environment
1. Enhance customer service excellence by making continuous improvement in the Press Ganey priority areas
2. Increase market share
3. Coordinate select clinical programs with YNHHS

Measures:
- Patient satisfaction continuous progress toward ≥ 90th percentile overall inpatient, maternity, ED
- BH "Most Preferred" score ≥ 29%
- Discharges > 20,025
- ALOS ≤ 5.25 days
- Overall market share ≥ 24%
- ED visits (treated and admitted) ≥ 63,500; clinic visits ≥ 49,267; SurgEase ≥ 7,000; MedEase ≥ 1,500; private referred ≥ 47,680; ACRM outpatient treatments ≥ 42,591
- Physician satisfaction baseline set
- Resident work hrs targets met
- > 100 patients/month on research protocols
- ED renovation/expansion program commenced

Strategic Dimensions — Financial performance

Strategies:

Meet operating, cash, and capital requirements by efficiently managing resources and focusing on enhancing revenue, cash, and philanthropy
1. Ensure profitability (increase revenue and control operating costs)
2. Enhance cash and short-term investment returns
3. Increase philanthropy to support capital needs

Measures:
- Operating margin BH ≥ 1.5%
- Days in AR ≤ 50.2
- Days cash on hand ≥ 50
- Pricing/contract compliance > $1,000,000
- ED capital campaign initiated
- Endowment and pension investment return within 1% of the Cambridge mean
- All bond covenant ratios met
- Supply-chain savings ≥ $780,000

Source: Used with permission from Bridgeport Hospital, Bridgeport, Connecticut.

This electronic scorecard allows managers to see their key performance indicators immediately, drill down for detailed analysis on some indicators, and benchmark their performance against other system hospitals as a way to identify performance improvement opportunities. This scorecard, which continues to evolve and grow over time, has become a very valuable tool for tracking real-time performance.

BALANCED SCORECARD CASE STUDY 2: LAKE REGIONAL

Lake Regional Health System[2] is a 140-bed community not-for-profit hospital located in the resort town of Osage Beach, Missouri. It has six primary care clinics, four rehabilitation therapy sites, three pharmacies, and a home health care. Because of its location on the Lake of the Ozarks, Lake Regional experiences two completely different operating seasons—the summer season, in which utilization is heavy, and the winter season, in which utilization is low. Thus, Lake Regional faces a number of issues experienced by other hospitals located in resort areas.

In 2001, Lake Regional set a three-year goal to achieve overall excellence at the state and national levels. The system chose to develop programs that could be recognized as excellent by both the Missouri Quality Award (MQA, see www.mqa.org) and the Malcolm Baldrige National Quality Award (see www.quality.nist.gov). Interestingly, although the MQA does not require hospitals to follow a balanced scorecard approach, Lake Regional decided that the scorecard was the best way to get the job done.

At Lake Regional, the balanced scorecard elements were a byproduct of the strategic plan, which was created with inputs from the board, medical staff, and administration. The plan allows the health system to determine the basic goals that need to be achieved. In producing the plan, inputs such as internal and external environmental scans were developed. Subsequently, long- and short-term themes were shaped while goals and stretch goals for the balanced scorecard success factors were determined.

In the first year of the balanced scorecard plan, Lake Regional determined the key elements of the scorecard, which are the starting goals for each indicator. The indicators were meant to be the critical success factors for the organization. At Lake Regional, only a few days elapsed between finalizing the strategic plan and setting the balanced score-card goals. The goals were given judgmental values based on review of trends over the past one to two years. At the same time, stretch goals were developed based on best-in-class benchmarks.

In the second year, Lake Regional still used the strategic plan to retain its focus. However, more emphasis was placed on best practices, both hospitalwide and departmentwide. During this year, Lake Regional devoted a substantial effort to customer service as defined by inpatient, emergency department, and outpatient satisfaction; patient loyalty; and physician outreach. Financial goals continued to be set by work groups.

In the third year, with the overall hospital and departmental goals remaining in effect, employee goals were developed. Lake Regional believed that to truly achieve success, employees must write personal goals related to the overall hospital and departmental goals. For example, in line with a patient satisfaction goal, a floor nurse's personal goal could be, "If pain medication is requested, I will get it to the patient within 15 minutes." To show its commitment, administration at Lake Regional required that the scorecard be discussed at all monthly depart-mental meetings. This allowed, for the first time, all employees to see the financial big picture as well as the other scorecard elements.

Table 4.4 represents the indicators that have been developed by administrators at Lake Regional. The table includes goals and stretch goals that symbolize the levels of success that the hospital expected to achieve in this time frame. The table also illustrates that Lake Regional took the time and effort to determine the most important indicators for its success and then developed the specific values that it wanted to achieve. In late 2003, at the end of its initial three-year journey of excel-lence using the balanced scorecard approach, Lake Regional was cho-sen as a recipient of the Missouri Quality Award.

This strategy worked for Lake Regional, and it can work for your organization. It takes knowledge of the balanced scorecard process, determination, and perseverance to succeed. Try it out. Your organiza-tion will be better off for the effort.

Jane learned about balanced scorecard techniques from one of her good friends, Laura Johnson, CFO of Memorial General, a larger hospital located several towns away from Pleasant Flats. While discussing some

TABLE 4.4 LAKE REGIONAL HEALTH SYSTEM'S BALANCED SCORECARD
GOALS

		Critical Success Factor		Stretch Goal	Goal
Financial	1.	Agency use	Year to date	$0	$776,000
	2.	% outliers	Annual	8%	10%
	3.	Long-term debt/total capital	Annual	40.1%	48.5%
	4.	Reserves	Annual	$35,700,000	$27,000,000
	5.	Days cash on hand	Annual	145	111.9
	6.	Return on assets	Annual	7.0%	3.9%
	7.	Operating margin	Annual	5.2%	1.1%
	8.	EBIDA*	Annual	14%	9.6%
	9.	Excess margin	Annual	6.8%	3.4%
	10.	Age of plant	Annual	9.4	9.1
	11.	Consolidated bottom line	Annual	$7,200,000	$3,500,000
Customers	1.	Overall satisfaction rate			
		• Inpatient	Monthly	94%	> 88%
		• Emergency department	Monthly	89%	> 86%
		• Ambulatory	Monthly	95%	> 94%
	2.	Patient loyalty rate			
		• Inpatient	Monthly	72.8%	> 50.2%
		• Emergency department	Monthly	62.6%	> 48%
		• Ambulatory	Monthly	67%	> 51%
	3.	Physician satisfaction rate	Monthly	80	78.5%
	4.	Community awareness (referral line calls)	Monthly	400	340
Internal Processes	1.	Medicare average time discharge to billing	Monthly	5 days	10 days
	2.	Completion % of projects	Annual	100%	100%
	3.	Community-awareness rate	Monthly	100%	> 95%
Learning and Growth	1.	Employee turnover rate	Annual	17%	19%
	2.	Vacancy rate	Monthly	8%	10%
	3.	Performance evaluation completion rate	Monthly	100%	95%
	4.	Employee satisfaction rate	Annual	2.00%	2.22%
	5.	FTE[+] per adjusted occupied bed	Year to date	5.24	5.97

* EBIDA: earnings before interest, depreciation, and amortization; [+]FTE: full time equivalent
Source: Used with permission from Lake Regional Health System, Osage Beach, Missouri.

financial outcomes, Laura described the methods her hospital had adopted to foster improvements in care, satisfaction, and financial performance.

Six months ago at Memorial, the board began receiving a set of metrics that included balanced scorecard categories. Prior to that time, the board was not made aware of many of the metrics used, nor had the context of the various elements of these indicators been explained to them. When the metrics were first presented, the board was stunned by the information, especially by the disparity between actual values and the benchmark medians.

According to Laura, "The good thing was that the hospital, in the following month, was able to narrow the gap in several of the line-item indicators. This closing of the gap continued over the next several months. In fact, we are now talking about moving our goals up to much higher levels. Using the balanced scorecard tool has been great all around."

Jane reported these findings to Jon. Not surprisingly, Jon immediately started working with his leadership group to determine Pleasant Flats's most important indicators, set appropriate goals, and begin monitoring results.

NOTES

1. Carolyn Salsgiver, senior vice president, planning and marketing, Bridgeport Hospital, Bridgeport, Connecticut. Personal interview with the author, September, 2004. Information on Bridgeport Hospital was obtained with permission.

2. Information on Lake Regional Health System was obtained with permission.

REFERENCES

Kaplan, R., and D. Norton. 1996. *The Balanced Scorecard*. Cambridge, MA: Harvard Business School Press.

Studer, Q. 2003. *Hardwiring Excellence*. Gulf Breeze, FL: Fire Starter Publishing.

PRACTICAL TIPS

☛ Use the balanced scorecard document as the first page of the monthly financial and operating statement report to the board. Recipients of this report can then easily determine if the various organizational goals are being met.

- Align the entire organization through the use of a vision, dimensions, objectives, and indicator measures approach.
- Adopt a scoring system that incorporates benchmarking outcomes with balanced scorecard elements. This system allows for an effective, easy-to-understand monitoring of results.
- For goal-setting and monitoring purposes, include any value outcomes being used by outside agencies to evaluate performance—for example, financial ratios developed by bond-rating agencies.
- Develop scorecard indicators at the department-manager level that are fully aligned with the overall balanced scorecard values.

CHAPTER FIVE

The Emerging Role of Six Sigma and Its Metrics Application

Jon Taylor was beginning to see some success with the newly adopted metrics orientation. Managers, directors, and vice presidents were paying greater attention to a number of outcome measures. Having set goals for financial ratios as well as established patient satisfaction percentiles and clinical outcomes/quality indicators for the operating managers using a balanced scorecard, Pleasant Flats was already experiencing partial improvements in a number of areas.

But Jon was still frustrated. Now that the improvements had begun, he was hungry for more, and faster, changes. He was getting closer to realizing his dream of running an outstanding medical center that would be recognized in its community as a true leader in the healing arts, a facility whose excellence was backed by independent and authoritative sources. "What will it take to get us there?" he asked the hospital's director of quality improvement, Jill Brown.

Jill, a former nursing director, had an answer: "I have been reading and hearing about a new method for improving outcomes based on metrics. It sounds a little bit like magic to me, but apparently it works. It has been used in other industries for close to 20 years, and there have been reports that it delivers phenomenal results. According to the articles I have been reading, a number of hospitals have already adopted it."

Jon was intrigued. "Well, what does it take to get going with it?" he asked. "If this is only half as good as it sounds, it is probably worth giving a try. Get me some information by next week and let's see if we want to do it."

P ICK AN AREA TO measure. Determine your actual values. Compare those values to benchmark percentiles. Find the gap between your current outcomes and the level you wish to attain. All of these elements amount to only following the first step of the five-step management process discussed in Chapter 1: set the appropriate goal.

The barrier to the movement from developing goals (Step 1) to creating action plans to achieve goals (Step 2) and implementing the action plans (Step 3) has often been the lack of a reliable business process. In this chapter, we examine a metrics-based management model, which is adopted from other industries, that is starting to be employed in the healthcare industry. This system is known as Six Sigma.

WHAT IS SIX SIGMA?

Six Sigma is a data-driven decision-making management process that is effective for reviewing existing processes and validating the credibility of the data used to make decisions. It uses statistical methods to *determine the level of errors within the management processes and the variability within each of the process steps.*

The Six Sigma process allows organizations to lower operating costs by

- eliminating waste, rework, and non-value-added process steps;
- providing tools and techniques for establishing accurate and effective measurement systems; and
- establishing a structure and discipline focused on clinical and nonclinical error reductions.

Six Sigma comes to healthcare with an impressive record of achievements in process improvements and financial results. The financial benefits to the four major *Fortune* 500 companies that adopted Six Sigma in the 1980s and 1990s—Motorola, GE, Honeywell, and Allied Signal—are significant. The savings as a percentage of revenue vary, from 1.2 to 4.5 percent. Those are significant percentages that go right to the organization's bottom line. For a hospital with $50 million in net revenues, for example, the savings would amount to between $600,000 and $2.2 million a year! The investment in the Six Sigma program is considerably less than that amount.

Figure 5.1 Sigma Designation

2 Sigma = 308,537 errors out of 1 million chances
3 Sigma = 66,807 errors out of 1 million chances
4 Sigma = 6,210 errors out of 1 million chances
5 Sigma = 233 errors out of 1 million chances
6 Sigma = 3.4 errors out of 1 million chances

The savings come in the form of decreased errors and reduction in the variability within process steps. The errors and variability are inherent in all processes. Some errors are only costly and time consuming. However, within healthcare, errors can result in the loss of life, as the industry has been told by the Institute of Medicine (Kohn, Corrigan, and Donaldson 2000) and by HealthGrades (2004).

In addition, variations in processes are inevitable. Healthcare delivery is a complex process involving diverse skills, different patient needs, and advanced technology. A high degree of variation makes it challenging to anticipate and manage results. The core Six Sigma concept focuses on reducing variation found in any process such as billing, physician practices, patient triage and treatment, or the way employees use technology. Variation also leads to patient dissatisfaction and drives up costs. If you can reduce human variation in a particular process, you can significantly reduce the amount of unacceptable outcomes or "defects." Eliminating defects one at a time greatly increases the level of efficiency. By completing the Six Sigma process, many organizations have already experienced a triple win: greater quality, cost savings, and satisfied patients.

Six Sigma is both a statistical designation and a performance target. Embedded in the Six Sigma credo is the concept of standard deviations around the mean. Six Sigma represents six standard deviations from the mean and indicates the number of errors available within process steps, depending on the sigma attained (see Figure 5.1). For example, an organization operating at a 6 Sigma level in a particular process only incurs 3.4 errors per 1 million opportunities or is virtually defect free. Similarly, an organization operating at the 4 Sigma level experiences 6,210 errors for every 1 million opportunities, which is a real problem if, for example, the process is surgeries in the operating suites. According to Mikel Harry and Richard Schroeder (2000), developers of the Six Sigma process at Motorola, most processes operate at between 3.5 and 4.0 Sigma.

THE SIX SIGMA PROCESS

Six Sigma brings a discipline and metrics to combat the errors and the process variability through a vigorous data-driven decision-making process. It is an advanced form of continuous quality improvement (CQI) and total quality management (TQM) concepts. It takes data you already have, derives information based on the data to determine operational outcomes, and provides results in a consistent format across projects. Six Sigma is more data and statistics driven than CQI and provides much better knowledge of results.

The hallmark of Six Sigma is its use of a systematic five-phase, problem-solving process called DMAIC:

D = define
M = measure
A = analyze
I = improve
C = control

DMAIC helps ensure that teams stay on track by establishing deliverables at each phase.

The DMAIC process begins by *defining* the problem as well as those items critical to quality (CTQ). Then, performance of those CTQs is *measured*. An *analysis* of the situation follows to find root causes of the problem and determine which problems have the most impact. With the causes identified, organizations can *improve* the situation by initiating change. The final step initiates measures to sustain the improvements that have been made for long-term *control*.

This systematic process is designed to dig in deeply, root out the problem, and ensure the solution is sustainable.

SIX SIGMA TERMS AND TOOLS

To use the Six Sigma process, the organization's leadership, management, and staff are required to learn new terms and rely on new tools in their business practices. Figure 5.2 is a listing of these terms and tools, which are not difficult to master and "turn managers into statistical thinkers," according to Nick Nauman, a Six Sigma black belt who has worked with many managers in the process.[1]

SIX SIGMA AND THE BALANCED SCORECARD

Combining the balanced scorecard performance indicators with the statistical rigor of Six Sigma can effectively focus an organization on the achievement of strategic goals. As stated by Bradley J. Schultz (2000) in his article "Merging Six Sigma and the Balanced Scorecard,"

> A Balanced Scorecard approach provides the mechanisms to drive organizational alignment, sustain improvements and maintain equilibrium across the enterprise. Based on statistics and aspects deemed most "critical to quality," Six Sigma could further focus the organization's improvement efforts. Such an approach that identifies and statistically quantifies the impact of causal factors on healthcare's value chain would provide organizations with a solid foundation for change.

Thus, any organization that decides to bring the balanced scorecard metrics approach together with the Six Sigma DMAIC process has an opportunity to achieve successes far in excess of successes that can be attained from following one of the methods alone. This prospect remains for many organizations that are currently practicing both management techniques and for those that are thinking about them.

SIX SIGMA IN HEALTHCARE

Since the late 1990s several hospitals and health systems have adopted Six Sigma. Its use in healthcare today is common, as more and more CEOs and COOs hear about the significant benefits that are available. Early adopters of Six Sigma relied on consultants from other industries. Chief executives were lured to the process after hearing stories that Six Sigma can significantly improve customer satisfaction and quality outcomes and can reduce costs. For example, early adopters Virtua Health in New Jersey and Valley Baptist Health System in Texas

FIGURE 5.2 SIX SIGMA TERMS AND TOOLS

- Control chart—method of monitoring variance in a process over time and alerting the business to unexpected variance that may cause defects.
- Critical to quality—element of a process or practice that has a direct impact on its perceived quality.
- Customer needs, expectations—as defined by customers, basic requirements, and standards.
- Defects—sources of customer irritation. Defects are costly to both customers and manufacturers or service providers. Eliminating defects provides cost benefits to the organization.
- Defect measurement—process for accounting for the number or frequency of defects that cause lapses in product or service quality.
- Pareto diagram—graph that focuses on efforts or the problems that have the greatest potential for improvement; shows relative frequency and/or size in a descending manner. This is based on the proven Pareto principle: 20 percent of the sources cause 80 percent of the problem.
- Process mapping—workflow description of how things get done, which enables participants to visualize an entire process and identify areas of strengths and weaknesses. It helps reduce cycle time and defects while recognizing the value of individual contributions.
- Root-cause analysis—study of original reason for process noncompliance. When the root cause is removed or corrected, the nonconformance will be eliminated.
- Statistical process control—application of statistical methods to analyze data and to study and monitor process capability and performance.

Six Sigma Positions

- Master black belt—Six Sigma teachers. They review and mentor black belts. Selection criteria for master black belts are quantitative skills and the ability to teach and mentor. Master black belts are full-time positions.
- Black belt—leaders of team responsible for measuring, analyzing, improving, and controlling key processes that influence customer satisfaction and/or productivity growth. Black belts are full-time positions.
- Green belt—similar to black belt but is not a full-time Six Sigma position. Often, these are managers of their own departments.

both enjoy the considerable savings that resulted from their Six Sigma utilization. Today, stories of success with this process abound ("Can Six Sigma Cure Health Care?" 2004).

SIX SIGMA CASE STUDY: COMMONWEALTH HEALTH CORPORATION

Commonwealth Health Corporation (CHC) was an early adopter of Six Sigma. CHC is the holding company for a diverse group of healthcare businesses headquartered in Bowling Green, Kentucky. It is made up of three acute care hospitals—the Medical Center at Bowling Green (with 330 beds), the Medical Center at Scottsville (with 47 beds), and the Medical Center at Franklin (with 25 beds). CHC also operates a specialty hospital (with 28 beds), billing service, credit agency, long-term care facility (with 110 beds), primary care clinic, large managed care network, home health business, laundry service, set of physician practices, and free health clinic. The corporation employs more than 2,500 employees and admits an average of approximately 16,000 patients per year.

In the 1990s, CHC's leadership decided to commit to a corporatewide Six Sigma process as an opportunity to drive major changes in the organization. John C. Desmarais, CHC's president and CEO, believes wholeheartedly in the power of the Six Sigma methodology and deemed the initiative "non-negotiable." According to Jean Cherry, executive vice president at CHC, "Certainly [Six Sigma's] ability to improve processes and make a tremendous difference in the way in which care is delivered makes it impossible to argue against its importance" ("Can Six Sigma Cure Health Care?" 2004).

According to Cherry, Six Sigma has made an impact on every aspect of CHC's operations. For example, errors in an ordering process dropped by 90 percent. Meanwhile, operating expenses in the same division were reduced by $800,000, and employee satisfaction rose by 20 percent. CHC followed up with an effort to improve the handling of diagnostic imaging. The cost per radiology procedure dropped by 30 percent, from $68.13 to $49.55. Based on 100,000 procedures, the cumulative savings exceeded $1.65 million. Errors in the MRI ordering process were reduced by 90 percent.

FIGURE 5.3 COMMONWEALTH HEALTH CORPORATION'S
CRITICAL-TO-QUALITY MEASURES

1. Quality of care/service
2. Customer satisfaction
3. Timeliness/speed/convenience
4. Cost

Source: Used with permission from Commonwealth Health Corporation, Bowling Green, Kentucky.

In February 2003, Desmarais announced the next phase of CHC's Six Sigma initiative. Cherry says this phase focused on the strategic alignment of projects and improvement efforts with organizational resources and corporate targets. "Our commitment was to increase the pace of improvements and the effectiveness of Six Sigma projects," says Cherry. "Commonwealth Health Corporation is charged to achieve very aggressive goals involving three critical areas of our organization: customer satisfaction, quality of service, and cost efficiency. Our executive vice presidents sponsor these metrics and continue to drive the improvements related to each." With its successful use of the process, CHC developed a Six Sigma vision: "By the year 2004, we will be proudly recognized by our employees, patients, clients, community, physicians and payors as the unquestioned leader in care and service, providing flawless quality never before achieved in the healthcare industry" ("Can Six Sigma Cure Health Care?" 2004).

As the core goal of leadership is to develop and communicate a vision, CHC's administration clearly demonstrated their skills. They determined those elements that were most critical to quality outcomes, which are known in Six Sigma terminology as CTQs (see Figure 5.3). These CTQs also represent the specific business objectives that need to be analyzed for each Six Sigma project.

To be the unquestioned leader in its field, CHC first needed to understand those measures that were important to all its customers and second to determine the benchmarks it needed to achieve to be the best. Only then could it operationalize the power of Six Sigma to help identify the action plans and the ways to implement the plans. CHC determined its customer expectations through a variety of means, including focus groups, surveys, interviews, and observations.

FIGURE 5.4 COMMONWEALTH HEALTH CORPORATION'S INITIAL
SIX SIGMA AREAS

Functional Service Areas
- Radiology
- Billing
- Admissions
- Documentation/charge entry
- Human resources/employment processes
- Managed care/staffing patterns

Clinical Service Lines
- Pulmonary-related illnesses
- Maternal care
- Surgery processes

Source: Used with permission from Commonwealth Health Corporation, Bowling Green, Kentucky.

Next, CHC statistically analyzed those areas that had the greatest opportunities for improvements. The areas chosen either had high cost, high utilization, or low quality. Figure 5.4 is a list of those initial areas targeted for CHC's Six Sigma projects.

Based on its CTQs, CHC's Six Sigma projects emphasized the following:

1. Customer service and satisfaction, as characterized by reduced wait times and consistent service
2. Quality of care, as characterized by reduced medical errors, increased patient safety, and the use of appropriate technology
3. Reduced cost, as characterized by increased productivity and reduced variations

Project Example: Women's Health Specialists

A prime example of one of CHC's projects using the Six Sigma process is an initiative undertaken to reduce patient wait times at the Women's Health Specialists practice. The process measured was from the time of arrival to the time of dismissal. As shown in Figure 5.5, baseline

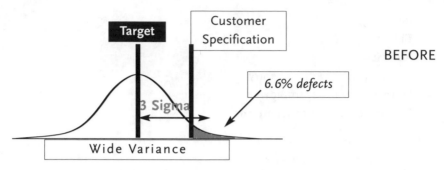

BEFORE

Defect: Any patient waiting beyond 60 minutes

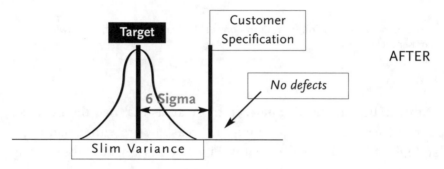

AFTER

Source: Used with permission from Commonwealth Health Corporation, Bowling Green, Kentucky.

analysis revealed that CHC's goal of moving patients through the system in under 60 minutes was designated at only a 3 Sigma level. Note that the 60-minute target established by CHC was the customer specification stated through patient surveys and focus groups. This baseline analysis also indicated that a wide variation in the patient flow existed, as characterized by the long length of the bell curve.

After CHC implemented some action plans to achieve its stated goal, several notable outcomes were revealed. The biggest outcome was that the shape of the bell curve dramatically thinned out, indicating a much smaller variation in the wait time for the patients. This reduction in variation led to more efficient use of resources, which was only one of the positive outcomes. Overall, this initiative had significantly positive effects on the operation of the Women's Health Specialists clinic.

FIGURE 5.6 CHC's Six Sigma DMAIC Process for Reducing
Inventory for Special Procedures and Intervention
Supplies

Define
- Identify customer specifications

Measure
- Collect data
- Create process map

Analyze
- Determine cost/benefit

Improve
- Ensure improvements are statistically valid and statistically tested

Control
- Prove the process is fixed and will not revert back to its original state
- Monitor cost/benefit

Source: Used with permission from Commonwealth Health Corporation, Bowling
Green, Kentucky.

Project Example: Inventory System

Using the Six Sigma approach, CHC developed a plan to reduce inventory for special procedures and interventional supplies. Figure 5.6 represents the steps taken to achieve results. By increasing inventory turns, improvements were made to the process. The CTQ business objectives were in the areas of cost and timeliness/speed/convenience. Two CHC Six Sigma black belts were chosen to assist the green belt (the department manager) assigned to the task.

In developing any Six Sigma project, it is imperative to define the defects in the processes that cause less-than-optimum outcomes. Reducing/eliminating these defects leads to the improvement of processes, the increase of Sigma level of quality, and the decline in variations. For this inventory-reduction project, a defect was defined as (1) any item in stock and not used (obsolete), (2) items with wrong item numbers, (3) items with wrong charge codes, and (4) items not charged (lost charges).

FIGURE 5.7 CHC'S BASELINE FLOWCHART FOR SPECIAL INVENTORY

Manual inventory completed once	Purchasing delivers supplies	Supplies are used for each exam
↓	↓	↓
Fill out order form for needed items	Supplies signed in and placed in inventory	Checkmarks are placed on charge sheet
↓		↓
Fill out internal record stock card		Sheet sent to hospital information
↓		
Department head signature on order form		
↓		
Fax form to purchasing		

Source: Used with permission from Commonwealth Health Corporation, Bowling Green, Kentucky.

Also as part of the Six Sigma methodology, the process that is being observed and improved must first be *measured*. In this case, measurement meant flowcharting the baseline process to determine the bottleneck points and areas for improvements. Figure 5.7 represents the baseline workflow created for this process. This flowchart shows a fragmented system, involving a lot of manual labor that causes a great deal of human error. For example, the second step in the process—fill out order form for needed items—presents opportunities for several errors to occur, such as writing the wrong item name, the wrong item number, the wrong quantity, or the wrong supplier. Multiple mistakes can occur with just this one process step!

Along with the flowchart, a supply inventory was performed. Data on the number and price of each item ordered within a 12-month period

FIGURE 5.8   CHC's Pareto Chart Showing Defects

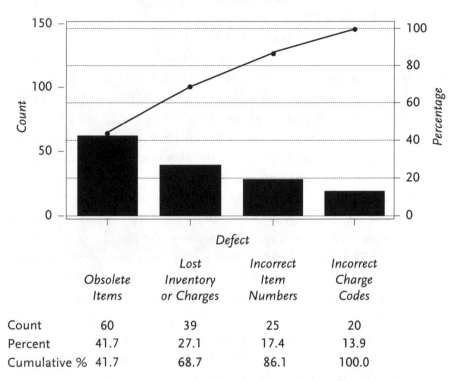

Defect	Obsolete Items	Lost Inventory or Charges	Incorrect Item Numbers	Incorrect Charge Codes
Count	60	39	25	20
Percent	41.7	27.1	17.4	13.9
Cumulative %	41.7	68.7	86.1	100.0

Source: Used with permission from Commonwealth Health Corporation, Bowling Green, Kentucky.

were obtained from the materials management department. To complete the comparative analysis, data on the number of items used (charged for) within the same 12-month period were also obtained from information technology. A data-collection tool (runchart) showed a discrepancy in the number of items ordered between the two sets of data because of incorrect items and charge numbers. With the use of fishbone diagrams and Pareto charts (see Figure 5.8), determining the magnitude of the defects was not difficult. Figure 5.8 illustrates that having obsolete items was the number-one reason for the defects, while the occurrence of lost charges was the second.

With this information at hand, the Six Sigma green belt (department manager) was able to develop the following improvements:

1. Obsolete items (items that are no longer used): there were 60 obsolete items (13 percent of the total inventory, or $30,791 in

value) in the special inventory. All obsolete items were removed from the inventory, and some items were exchanged for active inventory items. Other items were old and could not be returned for credit, so they were donated for educational purposes. The inventory no longer holds obsolete items.

2. Lost inventory or charges: automated inventory was implemented, and everyone in the department was made aware of the importance of properly charging patients for the items used. The automated inventory has significantly decreased the man-hours spent on doing inventory, filling out paperwork, generating purchase order numbers, and placing phone calls to order supplies.

3. Incorrect item numbers: the initial data collection revealed that 25 items had incorrect item numbers. Each item on the inventory list was verified with purchasing to ensure it had the correct item number. The item numbers on the 25 items were corrected, and the incorrect item numbers were deleted from the system.

4. Incorrect charge codes: the initial data collection revealed that 20 items had incorrect charge codes. Again, each item on the inventory list was verified with purchasing to ensure it had the correct charge code. The charge codes on the 20 items were corrected, and the incorrect ones were deleted from the system.

Additionally, the green belt was able to establish that improvements using the Six Sigma process were significant. During the initial baseline analysis, there were 107 documented defects out of a possible 288 opportunities. After the system redesign, however, there were 0 defects out of 229 opportunities, a remarkable achievement. This improvement was clearly the result of the change in the workflow. Figure 5.9 represents the process flowchart after the inventory system was redesigned and automated.

Financial Outcomes of Inventory Project

One of the ways Six Sigma goes beyond traditional CQI and TQM methods is in its use of positive financial outcomes. All Six Sigma projects must first go through a financial analysis before they are approved. This analysis should include projected improvements that must be certified by the finance department and then reviewed after the project is completed to determine if the projected financial outcomes were

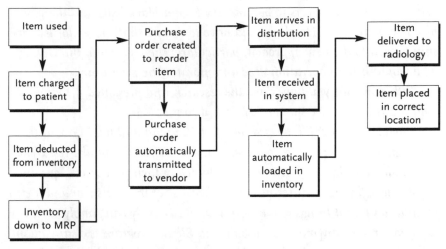

Source: Used with permission from Commonwealth Health Corporation, Bowling Green, Kentucky.

achieved. For this inventory project, the final numbers were presented as follows:

Lost inventory resulting in items not charged	$46,452
Incorrect charge codes resulting in overcharges to patients	7,408
Incorrect charge codes resulting in undercharges to patients	2,360
Total	$56,220

Different Six Sigma projects can have different financial outcomes. With the Six Sigma methodology, no level of financial improvement is prescribed for a project. After all, Six Sigma, like the balanced scorecard approach, has a variety of outcomes, some of which are nonfinancial. Six Sigma can and should be used by all healthcare organizations to achieve their goals.

Jon felt a little trapped after receiving information from Jill about the Six Sigma process. He had a decision to make, and he was not sure he wanted to make it. Six Sigma, despite all of its promised positive outcomes, sounded daunting and expensive to bring into the organization. It seemed to take a full-blown commitment and would undoubtedly change the entire culture of the organization, but for the better Jon knew.

Jon would have to convince the board, hire consultants, and train the better full-time managers to become Six Sigma black belts and therefore hire new managers. He also would have to ensure that the senior leadership buys into the new approach, particularly the COO and the CFO, who would help to operationalize and monitor the program.

"Jill, now that you have done the research and presented it to me, what do you think we should do?" asked Jon.

"Well, Jon," said Jill, "based on what I've read and heard about this Six Sigma program, it sure looks like a winner. Every hospital I researched has made marvelous strides in a whole bunch of their outcomes—quality, satisfaction, financial. It seems to work because of the statistical and metrics orientation that it brings to the organization. Nobody can simply get away with poor results anymore because the Six Sigma program is clearly quantifying the outcomes, which become easily comparable with the goals. I know that it will change our culture, and I have thought about this. But, you know Jon, our culture can use some change. You know that we are not achieving the kinds of results that you want. I do not think that Six Sigma is just a flavor-of-the-month program either. I think that the way it is set up will help Pleasant Flats to maintain it and produce enhanced results in the short term and the long term."

"Jill, I think you are right," said Jon. "Although it will change a lot in the way we manage, I think we need to do it. Please set up an action plan for me to take to the board and the senior management to move us down this road."

NOTE

1. Nick Nauman, Six Sigma black belt, Commonwealth Health Corporation, Bowling Green, Kentucky. Personal interview with the author, August, 2004. Information on CHC was obtained with permission.

REFERENCES

"Can Six Sigma Cure Health Care?" 2004. In 6L 1 (1): 1, 6–7.

Harry, M., and R. Schroeder. 2000. *Six Sigma: The Breakthrough Management Strategy Revolutionizing the World's Top Corporations.* New York: Currency Book.

HealthGrades. 2004. "Patient Safety in American Hospitals." [Online article; retrieved 6/1/04.] http://www.healthgrades.com/media/english/pdf/HG_Patient_Safety_Study_Final.pdf.

Kohn, L. T., J. M. Corrigan, and M. S. Donaldson (eds.). 2000. *To Err Is Human: Building a Safer Health System*. Washington, DC: The National Academies Press, Institute of Medicine.

Schultz, B. J. 2000. "Merging Six Sigma and the Balanced Scorecard." [Online article; retrieved 6/1/04.] http://healthcare.isixsigma.com/library/content/c031028a.asp.

PRACTICAL TIPS

☞ Research and read the Six Sigma methodology to determine if your healthcare organization is interested in adopting the process.

☞ Have a thorough discussion with your senior management to gain buy-in for the method.

☞ Contact consultants who specialize in Six Sigma implementation if you are not comfortable proceeding on your own.

☞ Implement many Six Sigma projects at one time (go for the big bang), or start slowly with two or three projects that are easily achievable and explainable (such as the shorter CHC project list in Figure 5.4). Smaller projects will pave the way for greater success with future Six Sigma initiatives.

CHAPTER SIX

Additional Clinical Metrics That Make an Impact on Operational Results

Jill Brown, Pleasant Flats's director of quality improvement, thought she was having a breakthrough year. Over the past several months, her boss (the CEO Jon Taylor) had been much more receptive to a number of her proposed initiatives involving the use of clinical outcomes and quality indicator metrics. She knew that Jon had been working toward adopting a new information-driven hospital strategy that involved the increased use of metrics. During her conversation with him, however, Jon had expressed concern with some of the metrics that she was proposing for clinicians at the organization.

"Jill, look," Jon said, "even though I am more convinced every day that the use of metrics is our future, and even though I really want Pleasant Flats to show real improvements in a number of the balanced scorecard measures we have adopted so far, I am a little troubled by the use of clinical and quality metrics. I have been getting a lot of heat from several of our leading physicians about the initial adoption of some of these metrics. They have not only been upset by the reporting of some of their outcomes for everyone to see but also by the benchmarking of those outcomes."

"Jon, I have heard many of the same things over the past few months," replied Jill, "but I have spent a lot of time explaining to many of these doctors the reasons that these clinical and quality metrics are so important. Some have listened, but others continue to resist the notion that measurement of their results and the hospital's is a good idea. In several cases, Jon, it seemed to make no difference to them that some of these metrics are being required by existing and upcoming government rules. I also explained to them that there are groups in the country that are able to collect our clinical and quality outcome information and compare us to our competitors. They didn't like to hear it, so they simply told me to stop using them!"

"Well," said an exasperated Jon, "you know that I have become a supporter of the use of metrics, but I also would like to keep our information private. We should be able to use it, but others should not be able to use it against us. Is there a way of making such information stop?"

"I can't stop it because we are not directly providing it," answered Jill. "These nongovernmental groups are getting it from legal sources. Meanwhile, state and federal governments are looking to report these results to the public. You know that the public has a right to know about our outcomes. But, Jon, there is a point here being missed by the doctors. They are so concerned about having their results reported because, at this time, their results are not favorable compared with their peers. Instead of trying to determine why their results are unfavorable, they blame the reporters. Remember, these clinical results have been severity adjusted to take into account the claim that their patients are sicker. With all due respect, I really believe that when they complain to you again about the reporting and comparing of their outcomes, you need to let them know that they need to find out how to improve. That is the whole point of the goal setting through benchmarks, reporting, monitoring, and feedback that you and I have been trying to instill in them this year."

"Jill, I know you're right. Still, it is easier said than done," sighed Jon. "We are on this road right now, and I want to finish our little journey. So show me again those clinical and quality measures that can help us greatly improve, and I will work with the doctors to try and move them along."

IN THIS CHAPTER, specific high-level clinical metrics will be emphasized. Many clinical metrics make a considerable impact on the organization's operational and financial results. Although these metrics may be familiar to some administrative personnel, they are often not distributed to those—management and staff alike—who can benefit from the information. For example, almost all clinical outcomes have an impact on financial performance; yet, in many hospitals, financial leaders, management, and analysts may not be aware of the clinical measures that are being collected and reported.

In seminar classes over the past five years, this author has surveyed hundreds of healthcare finance executives, managers, and staff. They revealed that very few of them had been exposed to critical clinical and quality outcome metrics collected by their organization. The reasons given for this deficiency are often the same: they were not aware that collection was taking place, and they were not aware of the contributions the results made toward the organization's financial health.

Further, little cross-pollination of clinical metrics was happening outside the clinical-operations areas of nursing, ancillary services, and physician leadership and outside the boardroom. Financial metrics were more likely to be shared across silos—generally at the executive and administrative levels—but clinical metrics were rarely shared.

The clinical and quality metrics discussed in this chapter have great applicability to the healthcare organization's balanced scorecard outcomes. Like all metrics described in this book, they should be shared, discussed, debated, and agreed on so that the organization can significantly improve its results. Again, the organization must do the following:

- Set appropriate and aggressive goals.
- Monitor the results of the actual values against the goals.
- Ensure that positive and negative consequences are in place when the goals are either being met or falling by the wayside.

THE JOINT COMMISSION'S METRICS INITIATIVES

Since the late 1980s, clinical metrics have been available for use in benchmarking, goal setting, operational improvement, and monitoring activities. The Joint Commission on Accreditation of Healthcare Organizations introduced the Agenda for Change in 1987. This agenda began the process of acknowledging the use of clinical metrics within the hospital industry. It included a set of initiatives designed to emphasize the importance of actual organizational performance in receiving accreditation. One year later, the Joint Commission introduced the Indicator Measurement System (IMSystem®)—an indicator-based performance-monitoring system (JCAHO 2004a).

Because the Joint Commission adopted the use of actual performance-based measures, hospitals around the country adopted a number of clinical metrics in the late 1980s and early 1990s. This allowed, for

Mortality
- Inpatient mortality
- Outpatient mortality
- Perioperative mortality
- Disease-specific mortality

Morbidity/Complications
- Infection control
- Hospital-acquired infections
- Surgical-wound infections

Utilization Statistics
- Rate of unplanned returns to the emergency room
- Rate of unplanned returns to the operating room
- Rate of C-sections
- Rate of vaginal births after C-sections

the first time, the development of benchmarking outcomes. Figure 6.1 shows a listing of some of the first clinical performance metrics that were implemented in the early 1990s. These clinical metrics set the stage for the many additional measures launched in subsequent years.

In February 1997, the Joint Commission launched its ORYX® initiative, which integrates outcomes and other performance measurement data into the accreditation process. ORYX®, implemented in phases for each accreditation program, is a flexible approach for supporting quality improvement efforts in JCAHO-accredited organizations. A component of the ORYX® initiative is the identification and use of standardized, or core, performance measures. In July 2002, hospitals began collecting core measure data on four initial measurement areas: (1) acute myocardial infarction, (2) heart failure, (3) community-acquired pneumonia, and (4) pregnancy and related conditions. The detailed performance metrics that apply to each of these four core measurement areas are listed in Figure 6.2.

In January 2003, hospitals began transmitting their measurement results to the Joint Commission. In July 2004, hospitals began collecting data on a fifth core measurement area: surgical-infection preven-

FIGURE 6.2 ORYX® CORE PERFORMANCE MEASURES (INITIAL SET)

Acute Myocardial Infarction
- Aspirin on arrival
- Aspirin prescribed at discharge
- ACEI* for LVSD**
- Adult smoking-cessation advice/counseling
- Beta-blocker on arrival
- Time to thrombosis
- Time to PTCA[+]
- Inpatient mortality

Heart Failure
- Discharge instructions
- LVF[++] assessment
- ACEI for LVSD
- Adult smoking-cessation advice/counseling

Community-Acquired Pneumonia
- Oxygenation assessment
- Pneumococcal screening and/or vaccination
- Blood cultures
- Adult smoking-cessation advice/counseling
- Pediatric smoking-cessation advice/counseling
- Antibiotic timing

Pregnancy and Related Conditions
- Vaginal birth after C-section
- Inpatient neonatal mortality
- Third- or fourth-degree laceration

*ACEI: Angiotensin-converting enzyme inhibitors; **Left ventricular systolic dysfunction; [+]Percutaneous transluminal coronary angioplasty; [++]Left ventricular failure

Source: The Joint Commission on Accreditation of Healthcare Organizations. 2004. [Online information; retrieved 6/04.] http://www.jcaho.org/pms/core+measures/information+on+final+specifications.htm.

tion. The Joint Commission is actively developing new measure sets that address intensive care unit care, pain management, and inpatient pediatric asthma. These measure sets are expected to become available incrementally between July 2004 and June 2006 (see www.jcaho.org/accredited+organizations/hospitals/oryx/the++next+evolution.htm).

Core Measures and the Accreditation Process

Each JCAHO-accredited organization is required to select core measure sets based on the healthcare services it provides. During the on-site survey, Joint Commission surveyors assess the organization's use of its selected core measure sets in its performance improvement activities. The Joint Commission inputs core measure data into a priority focus process to help determine onsite survey evaluation activities. The total number of measure sets an organization is required to use is relatively small. Individual organizations for which none of the core measure sets are applicable, based on their type of organization, continue to use their noncore measures to meet ORYX® requirements until applicable core measure sets are identified (see www.jcaho.org/accredited+organizations/hospitals/oryx/oryx+facts.htm).

According to the Joint Commission (2004b), "The goal of ORYX is to create a more continuous, data-driven, comprehensive and valuable accreditation process—one that not only evaluates a health care organization's methods of standards compliance, but the outcomes of these methods as well." Thus, the Joint Commission has made it an imperative for hospital administrators to establish a number of clinical metrics that affect the clinical outcomes of their patients.

Effectively, performance measurement in healthcare represents what is done and how well it is done. The goal is to accurately understand the basis for current performance so that better results can be achieved through focused improvement actions. Performance measurement is used by organizations internally to support performance improvement and externally to demonstrate accountability to the public and other interested stakeholders. Performance measurement benefits the organization by providing statistically valid, data-driven mechanisms that generate a continuous stream of performance information. This information then enables an organization to understand how well it is doing over time and supports its claims of quality.

Use of performance measures in healthcare allows an organization to do the following:

- verify the effectiveness of corrective actions,
- identify areas of excellence internally, and
- compare its performance with that of peer organizations that use the same measures.

Similarly, performance data can be used by external stakeholders in making value-based decisions on where to seek quality healthcare.

CLINICAL METRICS CASE STUDY: SSM HEALTH CARE

Among the processes that SSM Health Care[1] has developed to foster improvements at all levels of the organization is the use of clinical outcomes and quality indicators. As with any use of metrics, SSMHC leaders had to determine the specific measures that had the most impact on the organization. Interestingly, the mere act of determining these measures facilitated cross-pollination of ideas, which is helpful to organizational outcomes.

Table 6.1 illustrates several of the key measures that SSMHC has established for its clinical outcomes/quality indicator area. These measures are an offshoot of the key requirements that the organization established for its overarching objectives. The table shows that the established requirements lead to the key measures that then allow the organizational goals to be set based on benchmark information.

Within the care delivery/treatment measures in Table 6.1, SSMHC selected two metrics—percentage of congestive heart failure (CHF) patients receiving weighing instructions and percentage of ischemic heart patients discharged on proven therapies (Coumadin)—to show how it used goal development, benchmarking, and trend analysis to report its outcomes on the care delivery/treatment process category. The measure "use of dangerous abbreviations in medication orders" under the process pharmacy/medication use was also chosen to represent SSMHC's reliance on goal development, benchmarking, and trend analysis.

Figure 6.3 (page 126) specifically illustrates the method used by SSMHC to report the percentage of CHF patients receiving weighing instructions. By reporting the actual quality indicator percentages against the benchmark, SSMHC was able to adjust and improve its results. The reporting method for the percentage of ischemic (congestive) heart patients discharged on proven therapies is shown in Figure 6.4 (page 127). Once again, such reporting allowed the organization to move toward the benchmark goals.

As shown in Figure 6.5 (page 128), the percentage of medication orders using dangerous abbreviations not only indicates actual outcomes and the goals but also includes a benchmarking indicator. This allows

TABLE 6.1 SSM HEALTH CARE'S DELIVERY PROCESSES, REQUIREMENTS, AND MEASURES (PARTIAL LIST)

Process	Key Requirements	Key Measures
Admit		
Admitting/registration	• Timeliness	• Time to admit patients to the care setting • Timeliness in admitting/registration rate on patient satisfaction survey questions
Assess		
Patient assessment	• Timeliness	• Percentage of histories and physicals charted within 24 hours and/or prior to surgery • Pain assessed at appropriate intervals, per hospital policy
Clinical laboratory and radiology services	• Accuracy and timeliness	• Quality control results/repeat rates • Turnaround time • Response rate on medical staff satisfaction survey questions
Care Delivery/Treatment		
Provision of clinical care	• Nurse responsiveness • Pain management • Successful clinical outcomes	• Response rate in patient and medical staff satisfaction survey questions • Wait time for pain medications • Percentage of congestive heart failure patients receiving medication instructions • Percentage of congestive heart failure patients receiving weighing instructions (see Figure 6.3) • Percentage of ischemic heart patients discharged on proven therapies (Coumadin) (see Figure 6.4) • Unplanned readmissions/return to emergency department or operating room • Mortality
Pharmacy/ medication use	• Accuracy	• Use of dangerous abbreviations in medication orders (see Figure 6.5) • Medication error rate or adverse drug events resulting from medication errors

TABLE 6.1 *(continued)*

Surgical services/ anesthesia	• Professional skill	• Clear documentation of informed surgical and anesthesia consent
	• Competence/ communication	• Perioperative mortality • Surgical-suite infection rates
Discharge Case management	• Appropriate utilization	• Average length of stay • Payment denials • Unplanned readmissions
Discharge from care setting	• Assistance and clear directions	• Discharge instructions documented and provided to patients • Response rate on patient satisfaction survey

Source: Used with permission from SSM Health Care, St. Louis, Missouri.

the organization and its leaders to see the hospital with the best-practice outcomes. SSMHC provides a detailed trend-analysis chart to each of its hospitals' administration. This allows each hospital executive the opportunity to understand the facility's current outcomes, which in turn moves the executives to implement actions to achieve the facility's goals.

From a metrics analysis perspective, SSMHC has clearly spent the time to determine its most important clinical metrics. The corporation then requires a specific level of performance around each metric and provides a reporting mechanism that assists in periodically monitoring the progress toward goals. SSMHC is the epitome of an information-driven hospital. Its practices allow the system and its entities to excel in their efforts.

THE FUTURE OF CLINICAL METRICS

Clinical metrics that have been reported give a hospital valuable guidelines to follow; that is not enough, however. Each and every day, hospitals must continue to adopt and comply with the standards for collecting and reporting clinical metrics. Thus, they must also improve

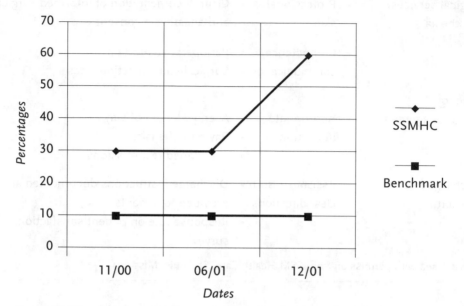

Source: Used with permission from SSM Health Care, St. Louis, Missouri.

the clinical outcomes they are generating. More and more healthcare and clinical quality organizations are taking clear steps to publish clinical data for public consumption. Thus, hospitals must take an aggressive role to ensure that they are achieving acceptable outcomes, as the information about their performance is increasingly made available.

For example, in 2004 the National Quality Forum (NQF) finalized two major reports related to clinical and quality measures. The first report, entitled "National Priorities for Healthcare Quality Measurement and Reporting," presents 23 NQF-endorsed priorities for healthcare quality measurement and reporting. These priorities cover the continuum of care and are organized into 2 infrastructure priorities, 5 process of care priorities, and 15 healthcare condition priorities. The highest priority across all of these areas is to reduce disparities in health and healthcare quality in vulnerable populations (NQF 2004a).

The second report, entitled "National Voluntary Consensus Standards for Nursing-Sensitive Care: An Initial Performance Measure Set," represents the first-ever set of national standardized performance measures to assess the extent to which nurses in acute care hospitals contribute to patient safety, healthcare quality, and a professional work

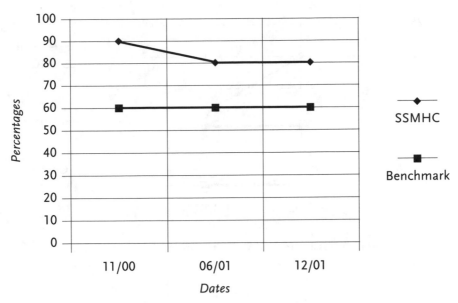

Source: Used with permission from SSM Health Care, St. Louis, Missouri.

environment. The measures of nursing care were sufficiently supported
by scientific data to gain the endorsement of various committees representing consumers, purchasers, researchers, providers, and health
plans. Measures include prevalence of conditions or events—such as
pneumonia, pressure ulcers, and falls—suffered as a result of a hospital stay. Other measures expand on this theme, such as the percentage of surgical patients who died after experiencing a complication
while hospitalized and the rate of pneumonia associated with the use
of ventilators in the intensive care unit. The standards also include
total work hours by nurses per 1,000 patient days (NQF 2004b).

The Leapfrog Group, the Centers for Medicare and Medicaid Services,
and the Joint Commission have all said they plan to incorporate NQF
standards in their quality-measurement efforts. Additionally, the Joint
Commission plans to make available to the public via the Internet the
performance information of JCAHO-accredited organizations. Termed
the Quality Reports, this publication includes information on an organization's accreditation status, accredited services, and compliance with

FIGURE 6.5 PERCENTAGE OF ORDERS WITH DANGEROUS
ABBREVIATIONS

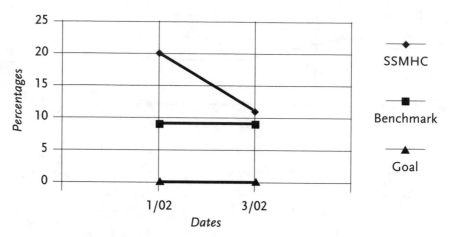

Source: Used with permission from SSM Health Care, St. Louis, Missouri.

the Joint Commission's National Patient Safety Goals and Quality Improvement Goals.

Finally, an article published on the front page of the *Wall Street Journal* in February of 2005 serves as another indicator that clinical benchmarking is in the future of U.S. hospitals, whether or not the healthcare industry is ready. The article highlights a specific campaign in Missouri that started with a single case of patient infection and ended with a law that requires hospitals in the state to gather and report their own nosocomial (hospital acquired) infection rates. Such legislative changes are being wrought around the country, and consumer groups are among the most active campaigners. Kenneth Kizer, president of the NQF, predicts that ". . . this [reporting requirement] will be universal before long" (Rundle 2005).

The future cries for more, not less, clinical outcomes and quality information. Hospitals must make the appropriate efforts to achieve and excel in these outcomes.

Jon was tired—tired of fighting with some of his managers, his administrators, and his board members about the new metrics-based, goal-oriented, results process that is rooted in accountability. Most of the organization, including the board, had gotten behind his move toward creating an information-driven hospital, but there were still some hold-outs. During a meeting with Jill, he expressed more of this exasperation.

"Okay, Jill, what can we do about some of these people who, for whatever reason, won't get on board with this new process?"

"It is a learning process, Jon," explained Jill. "Some people just learn slower than others. I know you want this complete buy-in, and I agree with you. But you have to decide if you want to pull the slow learners along or make an example of one of them by demoting or terminating their employment. If you choose the second option, it will become easy to determine which of the managers and division heads are not meeting and accepting the new goals that you set. You know that we have not had a culture of accountability until this year, and this process we are trying to implement would put an end to a lack of achievement by the management and our leadership group."

"Jill, that is a great idea!" exclaimed Jon. "I am going to call human resources right now and see just how I can go about doing this. Thanks for the advice. I knew you could help me."

NOTE

1. Information on SSM Health Care was obtained with permission.

REFERENCES

Joint Commission on Accreditation of Healthcare Organizations. 2004a. [Online information; retrieved 6/1/04.] http://www.jcaho.org/about+us/history/index.htm.

————. 2004b. [Online information; retrieved 6/1/04.] http://www.jcaho.org/accredited+organizations/hospitals/oryx/review+of+systems.htm.

National Quality Forum. 2004a. [Online information; retrieved 6/1/04.] http://www.qualityforum.org/webprioritiespublic.pdf.

————. 2004b. [Online information; retrieved 6/1/04.] http://www.qualityforum.org/txNCFINALpublic.pdf.

Rundle, R. L. 2005. "Some Push to Make Hospitals Disclose Rates of Infection." *Wall Street Journal* (February 1): section A, page 1.

PRACTICAL TIPS

☛ Develop clinical outcome and quality metrics that can be bench-marked. Set goals that move the organization from its current percentile up to and exceeding the 90th percentile.

☛ Share the results of the clinical metrics with administrators and managers outside of the clinical areas. This will allow for additional discussion on the meaning, contribution, and use of appropriate metrics.

CHAPTER SEVEN

Using Pay-for-Performance Models to Ensure Successful Action-Plan Implementation

Jon was feeling a whole lot better. As he reminisced about the year that was coming to an end, he realized that when the year started, Pleasant Flats Medical Center had been practicing a form of management best characterized by "gut." He now realized that the organization had not been using enough indicators and those used were often the wrong kind. Throughout the year, he learned to select and present those indicators that the organization's leadership group deemed most meaningful to achieving high quality, high satisfaction, and low cost.

In developing an improvement program, he had sought advice and assistance from his COO, CFO, and director of quality improvement. The four of them became a small committee that met on a weekly basis, and each week they hand-picked department managers to provide input. This group discussed issues throughout the organization. One week was devoted to nursing outcome measures, another week was allocated to overall ancillary quality measures, and other weeks were reserved for specific departmental outcomes such as for the imaging area, laboratory, cardiology, and so on. Some weeks were also spent addressing overall financial outcome measures and patient, employee, and physician satisfaction.

In all meetings, the managers made a presentation. The presentations always included a benchmarking component, wherein the presenting manager informed the executive team about the methods used to determine the appropriate indicators, the percentile ranks across a peer group, the selection of the peer group, the specific hospitals in the peer group, the actual indicator values at the organization in the previous 12 quarters, and the ways that peer hospitals were using the indicator to effect and/or monitor change. This format was a positive use of committee and management time and allowed the executive team to immediately determine whether to adopt the presented indicator for inclusion in either the departmental or organizational scorecard.

By year end, Jon and his executive team were able to take the next step in their development as an information-driven hospital. Through research, he learned that one way to effectively change the way the hospital was operating and to achieve substantially better results was to adopt a pay-for-performance package that extended from the CEO down to the staff members. The performance-pay initiative clearly defines to everyone in the organization the indicators that spell success for the hospital.

Now that the executive team had defined the indicators that were most meaningful for Pleasant Flats, Jon knew that it was time to put money where achievement was desired. In due course, he moved forward to implement the pay-for-performance technique.

O NE MODEL—PAY *for performance*—brings together most of the techniques that have been described in this book. It allows leadership to bring the bigger improvement strategies to smaller everyday practice of the staff.

Pay for performance is an incentive compensation technique that allows hospitals to do the following:

- Set specific goals, usually higher than budget (stretch goals).
- Monitor the results of the goals in an objective manner.
- Pay higher wages (or incentive compensation) based on the results.

The outcomes for performance are generally designed to reward achievements in a variety of balanced-scorecard-type areas such as quality, customer satisfaction, community, mission, projects, and finance.

Pay-for-performance outcomes can vary greatly, but they are specifically related to goals that have been set down by administration to achieve results. In fact, the intent behind this model is all about the numbers. The concept allows administration to reward those managers and staff who have shown a commitment to succeed on behalf of the organization. Additionally, it creates an organization that is all pulling in the same direction.

Because at least 3,000 hospitals are listed as tax exempt and not for profit, these organizations that want to adopt this pay system should seek legal advice so as not to violate any Internal Revenue Service Code 501(c)(3) regulations regarding private inurement. The likeliest way to prevent such problems is to ensure that financial results are not the sole criteria or even a major criterion in the payout methodology.

WHAT IS PAY FOR PERFORMANCE?

The employee-based pay-for-performance methodologies discussed here differ from another commonly named system used in healthcare. In the current environment, the federal government (through the Medicare program) and several managed care companies are beginning to adopt quality and outcome measures to determine whether to add or subtract reimbursement dollars, depending on quality results, to healthcare organizations. The reimbursement-based methodology is not covered in this chapter; however, the measures used by these third-party payers are likely to be used by healthcare organizations in setting metrics goals in the future.

The pay-for-performance methodology defined in this chapter was previously known as incentive compensation. The difference between incentive compensation and *pay for performance* is that the latter *brings specific value-added metrics down to the employee (associate) level*. Incentive compensation has been discussed, established, withdrawn, reestablished, reviewed, initiated, abandoned, dismissed, and reinstituted over the past 20 years. Initially, however, it was developed for senior leadership and later moved to the director and manager levels. Today, it is finally being used at the staff level in several healthcare organizations to assess and compel associate achievement.

In practice, pay for performance brings together all of the elements that make an information-driven hospital successful. The following two case studies delineate how pay-for-performance systems work.

Pillar	Plan Element	Maximum Points
Service	Customer service	15
Quality	Project management	35
People	Professional and staff development	20
Finance	Budget performance	20
	Management-discretion criteria	10
Total		100

Source: Used with permission from Sherman Hospital, Elgin, Illinois.

PAY-FOR-PERFORMANCE CASE STUDY 1: SHERMAN HOSPITAL

Sherman Hospital is a 353-bed hospital situated in Elgin, Illinois. In 2003, Sherman decided to adopt a new pay-for-performance methodology to improve performance. The system is tied to specific achievements based on objective metrics. The entire hospital has a number of goals, and these goals are applicable to everyone in the organization, from the CEO down to the entry-level staff member.

Sherman has adopted six pillars of success for its organization. Each of the pillars has specific measurable goals associated with outcomes. The pillars include superior service, high quality, best people, community outreach, volume growth, and financial performance. Different weights are given to different areas of the hospital. For example, service and quality are given a higher point weighting in the patient care areas than in the non-patient-care areas. Still, all divisions and departments need to achieve specific numerically based outcomes to share in the performance pay.

This case study shares an example of a specific department and the outcomes that are expected at Sherman. In this example, the information technology department is used to demonstrate the key elements of the plan and their maximum associated weights for performance pay. Table 7.1 represents the success pillars, the plan elements associated with the pillars, and the maximum points that can be achieved in the department to generate merit pay. Note that only four of the hospital's six pillars are represented in the table because the information technology department does not have any measurable goals associated with community outreach and volume growth pillars.

Included within the overall pillars and their plan elements are detailed scoring grids that allow for final scores to be tallied. For the information technology department, the components of each pillar paint an explicit picture of the important ingredients for success. Four elements are detailed below.

Service Pillar: Customer Service Element

- Annual information systems customer satisfaction survey score: *achieves target*
  - Baseline/fiscal year 2003 score: 3.23
  - Goal/fiscal year 2004 score: 3.37 (20 percent of one SD)
    » Score 3.37 or higher   10 points
    » Score 3.29–3.36 (* > 10 percent of one SD)   5 points
    » Score 3.15–3.28 (± 10 percent of one SD)   0 points
- Annual telecommunications physician satisfaction survey score: *achieves target*
  - Baseline/fiscal year 2003 score   2.92 points
  - Goal/fiscal year 2004 score   ≥ 2.50 points
    » Goal achieved   5 points
    » Goal not achieved   0 points
- **Total available customer service points**   **15 points**

Quality Pillar: Project Management Element

- Approved projects (or planned milestones in approved projects) are completed on time, within budget, and achieve a project survey score of 4 or greater (see Scoring Grid).
  - Achieve 90–100 percent project score   15 points
  - Achieve 75–89 percent project score   10 points

SCORING GRID

Project	On Time	Within Budget	Survey Score 4+
Project A			
Project B			
Project C			
Project D			
Project E			
Project F			
Project G			
Project H			
Project I			
Project J			
Project K			
Project L			
Project M			
Special Project 1			
Special Project 2			

- – Achieve 50–74 percent project score   5 points
- – Achieve < 50 percent project score   0 points
- Special projects (two) are completed on time, within budget, and achieve a project survey score of 4 or greater
  - – Maximum points   20 points
- **Total available project management points**   **35 points**

People Pillar: Professional and Staff Development Element

- 40 hours of professional development per year
  - – Exceeds target   10 points
  - – Meets target   5 points
  - – Does not meet target   0 points

- To effectively communicate with employees, at least 46 weekly staff meetings are held annually, at least 10 monthly department meetings are actively attended annually, and section meetings are attended as requested.
  - Meets target   5 points
  - Does not meet target   0 points
- Improve information systems and telecommunications employee satisfaction survey score on the question, "I enjoy working at Sherman Hospital."
  - April 2003 score for information systems   3.57 points
  - April 2003 score for telecommunications   3.89 points
    - » Goal achieved   5 points
    - » Goal not achieved   0 points
- **Total available professional and staff development points**   **20 points**

Finance Pillar: Budget Performance Element

- Information systems budgeted gross margin (before depreciation) of $XX; telecommunications budgeted gross margin (before depreciation) of $YY: *achieved*
  - Actual > 5 percent better than budget   20 points
  - Actual > 1 percent better than budget   10 points
  - Actual equals budget   0 points
- **Total available budget performance points**   **20 points**

Overall Financial Equation

Table 7.2 is the year-end pay-for-performance scorecard for the information technology department of Sherman Hospital. It includes the main categories of service, quality, people, and finance. As shown, points from the department's four pillars of success equate to percentages of increase for each individual staff member and manager of the department. The maximum points, based on the specified goals itemized above, are 90. Additionally, 10 more points are available at management discretion, which is based on a number of subjective criteria.

Pillar	Plan Elements	Maximum Points	Score Achieved	Points Awarded
Service	Customer service	15	3.14	0
	Information system customer satisfaction survey	10		
	Telecommunications physician satisfaction survey	5	2.39	0
Quality	Project management	35	see Table 7.3	
	Main projects	15	28 of 29	15
	Special Project 1	15	Achieved	15
	Special Project 2	5	Achieved	5
People	Professional and staff development	20		
	40 hours of professional development	10	40	10
	46 weekly staff meetings	5	46	5
	Improve employee satisfaction score:	5		5
	• Information technology		4.29	
	• Telecommunications		4.18	
Finance	Budget performance	20	> 7.5%	20
	Management discretion	10	Achieved	10
Total		100		85

Source: Used with permission from Sherman Hospital, Elgin, Illinois.

Achieving 100 points equates to 100 percent of the available merit opportunity (i.e., the maximum percent increase).

The increases are prorated based on the number/percent of points earned. For example, if the maximum merit possible is 4 percent and the department achieves 100 points, the staff members in the department are eligible for a 4 percent increase. Similarly, if the department achieves 50 points, the staff would be eligible for a 2 percent increase. The maximum percent increase is set each year through the budget process, and staff are told what the maximum is before the year begins.

As seen in Table 7.2, for the fiscal year ended in 2004, the information technology department achieved a total of 85 points. The merit-based performance pay awarded to the staff in the department was 85 percent of the 5 percent maximum award level, or 4.25 percent. This includes the information included in Table 7.3—the information technology project scorecard—that details the entire project management goals and achievements.

According to Barbara Mills, the chief information officer of Sherman Hospital,[1]

> By utilizing the IT balanced scorecard, we learned some lessons about customer satisfaction surveys, measuring success of projects, "incenting" staff based on the employee satisfaction survey, and approved variances from budget that we incorporated into the new score sheets for fiscal year 2005 (which started in May 2004). The bottom line is this process worked for IT last year and should work even better this year, now that we have one year under our belt. The staff is now much better informed and understands why their pay is adjusted the way it is. This has been a very useful technique.

PAY-FOR-PERFORMANCE CASE STUDY 2: CENTEGRA HEALTH SYSTEM

Centegra Health System[2] is a 338-bed system in McHenry, Illinois. It has more than 3,000 employees, 19,000 discharges, and 55,000 emergency department visits each year. It is an information-driven hospital that has developed a tradition of doing extremely well in metrics-based awards systems. By setting high goals around patient and family satisfaction, employee satisfaction (workforce commitment), and clinical outcomes, Centegra has been able to show its dedication to its community.

For example, in 2003 Centegra was recognized by the Loyalty Institute of Aon Consulting for making the most significant increase in the Workforce Commitment Index (WCI), a score that measures employee commitment and job satisfaction. The WCI is based on more than seven years of research in which questions were developed to measure and compare employee commitment on a national level. The measurement tool focuses on team productivity, employee pride in the

TABLE 7.3 SHERMAN HOSPITAL'S INFORMATION TECHNOLOGY PROJECT SCORECARD

Project	On Time	Within Budget	Survey Score 4+
Project A	1	1	1
Project B	1	1	1
Project C		Deferred by user	
Project D	1	1	1
Project E	1	1	1
Project F		Canceled by management	
Project G	1	1	0
Project H	1	1	1
Project I	1	1	1
Project J	1	1	(In process)
Project K	1	1	1
Project L	1	1	1
Project M		Delayed by vendor	
Special Project 1	0.8	1	1
Special Project 2	1	1	(In process)

Regular Project score: 28 of 29 points = 97%   15 points
Special Project 1: 2.8 of 3 points = 93%   5 points
Special Project 2: 2 of 2 points = 100%   5 points

Source: Used with permission from Sherman Hospital, Elgin, Illinois.

organization and its services, and employee intention to remain with the organization.

One of the ways that Centegra was able to achieve this award was in its use of a pay-for-performance methodology that focuses the staff and management on those issues most important to the health system's mission. In mid-2003, Centegra's CEO, Michael Eesley, sent a memorandum to every associate outlining a modified pay-for-performance system. As can be seen in Appendix 7.1, the system was designed to move the managers and their associates into new areas of substance for the organization.

The memo (see Appendix 7.1 on page 145) clearly outlines the value-added focus areas for the hospital in the upcoming year. It further clarifies exactly how the program will work and presents examples so that the associates can clearly appreciate what the program will mean to them. Pay for performance is an excellent technique for addressing the essential needs of the organization. It is the best, most positive, and most understandable method for moving this system or any other hospital or healthcare organization forward in adopting goals and achieving outcomes.

Additionally, the pay-for-performance system *aligns* organizational needs with recognizable monetary results at the ground level. It brings together all of the elements of an information-driven hospital, starting with the selection of those numeric goals that drive the organization's outcomes. The implementation of a pay-for-performance system will give any organization the best chance for success in its endeavors.

At the end of the first full year, Centegra was able to report very reasonable results from its pay-for-performance initiative. Table 7.4 details the actual results achieved in relation to the set goals along with the scoring weights associated with each initiative/priority. As shown in the last column, Centegra achieved a weighted score of 59 percent for the year. This score equated to a 3.11 percent pay-for-performance award, out of a possible 6 percent, for Centegra associates. Although only in its first year, the program made associates excited about the new initiatives and rewards.

When announcing the results of this pay-for-performance system in the first year, Centegra's administration took the opportunity to announce the second-year goals. Table 7.5 shows the goals set for fiscal year 2005. These goals reflect the outcomes of the 2004 results as well as the goals the administration requires for the following year. Thus, the initiation of a pay-for-performance system creates an ongoing and long-term metrics-based management technique that allows for a greater degree of accountability from all employee levels of the organization.

The two hospital systems featured in these case studies—Sherman and Centegra—have clearly demonstrated how to operationalize an

TABLE 7.4 CENTEGRA HEALTH SYSTEM'S FIVE STAR PLAN: CORPORATE PRIORITIES FOR THE 12 MONTHS ENDING JUNE 30, 2004

Corporate Priorities	Minimum (1%)	Target (50%)	Maximum (100%)	Weight	Score	Percent Achieved	Weight x Percent Achieved
1. Quality: Percent of complaints per Press Ganey	7.5%	7.2%	6.9%	0.10	5.4%	100%	10%
2. Finance: Year-to-date margin	$6,100,000	$8,595,500	$11,091,000	0.30	$7,042,200	18.9%	5.7%
3. People: Employee turnover	16.2%	14.6%	13%	0.15	13.6%	81.3%	12.2%
4. Growth: New service initiatives	$0	$2,964,000	$5,925,000	0.15	$1,498,944	25.3%	3.8%
5. Community: Press Ganey scores	65.0	77.0	87.0	0.30	85.0	90.9%	27.3%
			Totals:	1.00		Section score:	59%

Reconciliation

Section score from chart	59%
Maximum award	6%
Award based on performance	3.54%
Operating margin factor	87.86%
Actual award	**3.11%**

Source: Used with permission from Centegra Health System, Woodstock, Illinois.

Star	Value	Minimum	Target	Maximum
Quality	15%	80%	90%	100%
Finance	25%	2.2%	3.1%	4.0%
People	25%	89.4%	91.0%	92.6%
Growth	15%	0%	2.2%	4.4%
Community	20%	80.1	85.1	90.1

Source: Used with permission from Centegra Health System, Woodstock, Illinois.

information-driven hospital using metrics to drive achievement and success.

The pay-for-performance technique presented in this chapter is just one of several methods that can improve the outcomes of many American hospitals. This technique also offers a great opportunity for all levels of management and leadership (from the board chair to the department manager to the staff associate) to contribute to the overall goals of the organization. Pursuing it is definitely worth the effort, the time, and the inherent changes (and conflicts) that will occur.

Jon's year was over. In this brief span of time, Pleasant Flats had begun the transformation that so many hospitals are now embarking on—to become an information-driven hospital. In speaking with Jane Zabrowsky, his CFO, Jon marveled at the changes the organization has already carried out.

"Jane, it is amazing. We have sure come a long way," Jon commented. "I was just thinking about one of the smaller changes that we made when you cut down the size of the monthly financial package yet dramatically increased the really important information that we needed to manage this place. I appreciate your commitment to the process because you have certainly been a leader. You and Jill have certainly stepped up this year."

"Jon, thanks for the nice words. I know what you mean," replied Jane. "The improvements are so obvious to everyone, including the community leaders that sit on the board. They keep calling me to thank me for the changes. But the comments I like best come from the managers. They are

thrilled to finally have information that is meaningful to them, allowing them to actually manage the issues that we say are important. They have never been more alert to the differences between our expectations and their actual outcomes. It has brought calm to many of the processes that used to be a lot more chaotic. I sure am glad that you decided to commit to this information-driven hospital strategy."

"You know, so am I," said Jon. "This has been one of the best years that I have ever had as a CEO. And I plan to tell everyone I know about the ways that the successes were achieved. I am sure a convert to the process."

NOTES

1. Barbara Mills, chief information officer, Sherman Hospital. Personal interview with the author, October, 2004. Information on Sherman Hospital was obtained with permission.

2. Information on Centegra Health System was obtained with permission.

PRACTICAL TIPS

☞ Determine how much benefit a pay-for-performance model would bring to your hospital. As long as its benefits exceed the costs, such a model would add value to the organization.

☞ Ensure that the indicators used in the pay-for-performance system are aligned with the overall organizational goals. Performance pay gives recipients an incentive to achieve not only their own goals but those of the organization.

To: Centegra Associates   July 25, 2003

From: Michael S. Eesley
         President & Chief Executive Officer

RE: Our New Results-Sharing Plan Called the Five Star Plan

Centegra Health System has provided a Results Sharing Plan (RSP) since 1998. From this plan, monetary awards ranging from 0% to 3.9% of annual salaries have been paid out to Associates. Many individuals have voiced how complicated the RSP model is to understand, and due to the complexity, they had difficulty understanding how to impact these awards. For many of these reasons the Results Sharing Plan was carefully reviewed and the Five Star Plan was developed. This letter outlines our new plan.

The Five Star Plan focuses on performance measures developed around five key areas: Quality, Finance, People, Growth and Community. These areas are called the Five Stars of Excellence.

The Five Star Plan provides annual, performance-based, lump-sum cash awards to Associates. The principal goals of the plan are to:

1. Support and reward the achievement of mission critical organization-wide goals.
2. Focus our attention on the performance measures and goals important to CHS's viability and success.
3. Allow us to share in the success of CHS and its operating entities.

The Financial Threshold must be met in order for a payout to occur. After the minimum financial goal is met, awards will be based on the percent of each goal achieved. The five corporate priorities for FY2004 developed around the Five Stars of Excellence are outlined below:

CHS's financial threshold for FY2004 is the achievement of a 2.2 percent system-wide operating margin.

FY2004 CORPORATE PRIORITIES

1 Corporate Priorities	2 Minimum (1%)	3 Target (50%)	4 Maximum (100%)	5 Weight	6 Performance Achieved	7 Percent Achieved	8 Col. 5 x Col. 7
1. Quality: Percent of complaints per Press Ganey	7.5%	7.2%	6.9%	0.10			
2. Finance: Operating margin for system	2.2%	3.1%	4.0%	0.30			
3. People: Employee turnover	16.2%	14.6%	13.0%	0.15			
4. Growth: New service initiatives	$0	$2,964	$5,925	0.15			
5. Community: Press Ganey scores	65	77	87	0.30			
			Totals:	1.00		Section Score:	0.___

DEFINITIONS OF THE FIVE CORPORATE PRIORITIES

1. Quality: Percent of customer complaints from the Press Ganey patient satisfaction surveys—If 50 patients respond to the survey and there are 3 complaints, the percentage is 3/50 or 6%.
2. Finance: Operating margin—The money we receive from all payors, less the money we spend to cover salary, benefits and other bills. (This is like our checkbook balance.) The dollar amount that is remaining is translated into a percentage, which measures our financial health.
3. People: Associate turnover—When Associates leave Centegra and new Associates are hired to replace those positions, it is costly, disruptive, and can impact the quality of care. Therefore, the lower this percentage is, the better.
4. Growth: New service initiatives—New business is good for Centegra. It keeps us focused on providing the much needed services to our community.
5. Community: Press Ganey survey scores—This is a measure of patient satisfaction and the quality of care provided. The highest quality of care is our most important goal at Centegra. It is the average of the 15 surveys we send out.

An example of an award calculation for an Associate with annual FY2004 earnings of $35,000 is listed below.

Five Stars	Weight	Performance Achieved	Col. 2 x 3
Quality—Complaints/surveys	0.10	0.75	7.5%
Finance—Margin	0.30	0.50	15.0%
People—Turnover	0.15	0.50	7.5%
Growth—New business	0.15	0.50	7.5%
Community—Patient satisfaction	0.30	0.50	15.0%
		Sum	**52.5%**

Maximum award	6% or $2,100
Award amount	6% x 52.5% = 3.15%
Annual earnings	$35,000
Award amount	x 0.0315
Actual award	$1,102.50

WHAT HAS CHANGED?

The chart below provides a highlight of the Five Star Plan along with a comparison to the old Results Sharing Plan.

(continued on following page)

Category	Five Star Plan Beginning 7/1/03	Results-Sharing Plan (Past Model)
Eligibility	• Work a minimum of six months • Associate (excludes physician and contract employees) • Must be employed at the time of payout	• Active Associate • Same • Must be employed at the end of the fiscal year
Maximum awards	• Up to 6% • Excludes unproductive hours (i.e., ATO)	• Determined by performance indicator results
Plan funding and threshold performance	• Must achieve minimum financial threshold	• Must achieve operating margin and patient satisfaction
Corporate priorities	• Quality • Finance • People • Growth • Community	• Have ranged from four to twelve Key Performance Indicators
Performance measures	• Measures are indicated based on positive results	• Measures were indicated as both positive and negative results
Organizational structure	• Associates will receive award based on the corporate priorities	• Associate awards based on System and Division priorities

Look to your leaders to begin the discussion regarding the new Five Star Plan and how you can work as a team to impact the Five Star Plan. If you have questions regarding the Five Star Plan, you should discuss them with your leader. The new Five Star Plan will also be discussed at the Open Forums the week of July 28th.

Source: Used with permission from Centegra Health System, Woodstock, Illinois.

About the Author

Steven Berger, CPA, CHE, FHFMA, is president of Healthcare Insights, LLC, a firm that specializes in providing healthcare financial and general management training. Healthcare Insights developed INSIGHTS, a management accountability and decision-support software solution for the healthcare industry.

Mr. Berger has 30 years of healthcare financial management experience. Prior to his current role, he was vice president of finance at Highland Park Hospital in suburban Chicago. Before that position, he served as finance officer for several hospitals and health systems in New York, New Jersey, and Missouri.

Mr. Berger is a certified public accountant and holds a bachelor of science degree in history and a master of science degree in accounting from the State University of New York at Binghamton. In addition, he is a Fellow of the Healthcare Financial Management Association, for which he has served as president of the First Illinois Chapter, on the National Board of Examiners, and as the regional executive of Region 7. Mr. Berger is also a Diplomate of the American College of Healthcare Executives (ACHE).

Over the past several years, Mr. Berger has led or been a presenter for many healthcare finance seminars held throughout the United States and Canada. He also teaches a two-day class for ACHE called "The Information-Driven Hospital," from which this book is derived.

Mr. Berger has written or cowritten articles and books on healthcare financial and general management issues. His writing has appeared in well-respected publications such as *Healthcare Financial Management* magazine and *Modern Healthcare*. In addition, he is the author of *Fundamentals of Healthcare Financial Management*, which is now in its second edition (published by Jossey-Bass in 2002); is the author of *Understanding Nonprofit Financial Statements* (published by BoardSource in 2003); and is the coauthor of *Introduction to Hospital Accounting, 4th edition* (published by Kendall Hunt for HFMA in 2002).